DO YOU KNOW WHAT YOU DON'T KNOW. . .

ABOUT WOMEN'S HEALTH ISSUES?

CINDY A. KRUEGER, M. P. H.

Copyright © 2005 by Cindy A. Krueger M.P.H.

Published by
BC Publishing
4213 Sylvan Ramble St., Suite 100
Tampa, FL 33609

This book or parts thereof may not be reproduced in any form, stored in a retrieval system or transmitted in any form by any means; photocopy, mechanical, electronic, recording or otherwise, without prior written permission of the publisher, except as provided by United States of America copyright law.

This book contains information from research literature, experienced healthcare professionals, and scientists. It is not intended to provide medical advice or to take the place of your personal physician. Readers are advised and encouraged to consult with a healthcare professional for personal medical issues. Diligent efforts have been made to assure the accuracy of the information contained in this book as of the date of publication. The publisher and the author disclaim liability for any medical outcomes that may occur as a result of applying the methods suggested in this book.

ISBN: 0-9765542-0-8

Library of Congress Control Number: 2005902957

Cover design: Ann R. Griffin
Interior design: BudgetBookDesign.com

Printed in the USA

DEDICATION

THE WORK IN THIS BOOK is dedicated to John R. Lee, M.D., my good friend and confidant, who suddenly passed away October 17, 2003. Dr. Lee taught me about the therapeutic value of natural progesterone crème after I had suffered for years from severe menstrual cramping. He thoughtfully explained how to use it and why it was the safest and best intervention that replicates natural hormones in a women's body. It is a miraculous hormone that has changed my life forever.

He will always be remembered for his dedication, integrity, scientific expertise and commitment to women's healthcare issues. Because of his pioneering spirit and desire to uncover the truth, he brought the world of science to women in a simplistic manner that has changed and improved millions of lives.

At dinner one evening during one of his many visits to Tampa, Florida, I jokingly asked him what we, the world of informed women, would do without him when he died. He replied, *"You have all the information you need in my books. Go out and share it with the world."*

So here you have it. This book is just a small piece of what I have learned and researched and want to share with women so they will become informed about personal healthcare issues in order to experience a vital and energizing life. I am forever grateful for John R. Lee, M.D., a great and kind soul of the 21st Century.

As Saint Thomas Aquinas wrote: *"The greatest kindness one can render to any man consists in leading him to the truth."*

ACKNOWLEDGEMENTS

THIS BOOK IS THE CULMINATION of many years of experience and input from several mentors, friends and professionals. Without the gentle nudging from my patient and loving husband Bob, who I consider to be the salt of the earth, this project would not be complete. He kept me focused and on track to accomplish my goal and to make it happen in a timely fashion.

My brother Tom, a father of seven well-rounded, independent thinking children, has written a book, so if he had time to write one, I knew I could too. He also shared writing experiences and resources that have been invaluable.

I am ever so grateful for Ann Griffin, my design artist, who is a beautiful gentle soul and an extremely talented woman in the field of design. She encouraged me to get the "truth" out to women and put it in book form. Without her guidance and talents, heaven knows what the cover of this book would have looked like.

I am blessed to still have my parents with me; they are now in their eighties. Everyday, they would ask me when this book would be complete. They are the true test of time in that they have engaged in very healthy lifestyle behaviors for many years. They are an inspiration to me and others and have always encouraged me to never stop learning and loving.

I would like to thank my friend Nancy, who planted one of the first seeds by encouraging me to write a book. Her encouragement and connections have been a great inspiration and support to me.

My heartfelt appreciation goes out to my editor, Beth Bruno, and my printer Books Just Books and Budget Book Design who assisted me in the final days of this project. I'm deeply appreciative for my dear friends and colleagues, Magda, Gay, Alyce, and Tom who gave up precious time with their families to review my manuscript. I am forever grateful for their literary expertise and comments.

Finally, my golden retriever Sadie laid by my side daily, reminding me to walk her and stretch out from behind my desk. She never failed to walk up to me and stick her nose under my arm for a little attention before going back to find a comfortable spot on the floor in the midst of scattered papers and journals to do what she does best...sleep. I have learned a great deal from this beautiful animal.

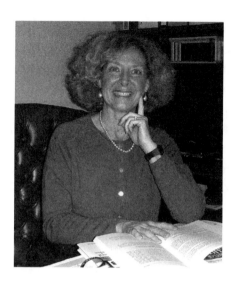

ABOUT THE AUTHOR

CINDY A. KRUEGER, M.P.H., is a health researcher with over 25 years experience in the healthcare industry. She is Founder and President of Preservion, Inc., a health information research, consultation and education company. Her professional experience in healthcare started at the Cooper Clinic Aerobic Center in Dallas Texas, noted throughout the world for its expertise in preventive medicine.

In the 1980s and 90s, she was the driving force in bringing preventive medicine concepts and programs to the Southeast's largest telecommunications company. Her expertise is designing preventive healthcare initiatives and strategies. She advises and counsels individuals and companies about healthcare choices and options using the latest research and scientific literature. She is published in *Driving Down Health Care Costs – Strategies and Solutions* and authors a monthly article for www.preservion.com

Cindy A. Krueger brings a dynamic and passionate message to professional conferences and organizations throughout the USA. Her regular guest appearances on television and radio empower consumers with scientific evidence supporting integrative and wholistic healthcare practices that help people live better, longer and more active lives.

She holds a Bachelor of Science (BS) degree in Physical Education and Health from the University of Southern Mississippi and a Masters of Public Health (MPH) from the University of South Florida.

CONTENTS

FOREWORD

SINCE RELOCATING TO TAMPA FLORIDA a couple of years ago, I have been fortunate to meet numerous health professionals who are passionate about helping others obtain good health in a more natural way. Physicians who have been conventionally trained in surgical specialties, internal medicine and family practice are just beginning to recognize that our current model of medicine is based on the premise of suppressing and treating symptoms and disease rather than true prevention, health and healing.

Innovative and clinically validated pathways to improved health are making their presence known through evidence-based outcomes in Integrative Medical Clinics across the country. Consumers today are becoming more educated, more proactive, and more accepting of the responsibility for their own healthcare. It is refreshing and exciting to witness the steps many enlightened individuals are taking to achieve a more wholistically minded approach.

I have been blessed in my 20-year medical career to experience a varied background, from my early days in pharmaceutical sales and marketing with Wyeth and Merck, to conventional family practice medicine and then transitioning into non-invasive natural therapies as a board certified naturopathic physician. More recently, the journey has included research and clinical trial experience utilizing natural medicines, including Natural Hormone Replacement Therapy (NHRT).

We are all being exposed to an environment with xeno-estrogens/xenohormones (environmental compounds that have potent estrogen-like activity not found in nature), that force the young female body into early puberty, thus impacting and disrupting the hormonal balance of women from an early age. Due to this change, more women today are taking control of their health and healing options. The perspective they bring through greater experience, discernment and evaluation enriches their pathway to a healthy life.

Meeting my good friend Cindy Krueger was, I believe, by design and not purely coincidence. We met on a late Friday afternoon at the University of South Florida, College of Medicine, Department of Public Health, where monthly Holistic Grand Rounds are held to discuss the model and future of *"good medicine"*. This is an informal monthly gathering of wholistically minded professionals who share their clinical and professional experiences and discuss natural approaches and therapies for chronic illnesses, diseases and conditions.

The focus of this *"good medicine"* is health, healing and education, which is emphasized throughout the pages of this book. In all my years in this industry, I have not met anyone with the integrity, ambition, and passion that Cindy has demonstrated to get the truth and the answers to women. Science-based data, such as the results from the Women's Health Initiative (WHI) and the Million Women Study (MWS) in the United Kingdom, supports the current trend toward bio-identical hormones and recommending micronized progesterone, USP, to achieve optimal health and wellness for perimenopause, menopause and beyond. These studies have also confirmed that the use of synthetic hormones is causing more risks and harm (heart disease, stroke, pulmonary embolisms and cancer) than benefits.

Other major changes in women's health have occurred over the last 10 years, including the entry of the term "estrogen dominance" (coined by John R. Lee, M.D.) into mainstream conventional medicine. The causes, symptoms and dangers of estrogen dominance were originally demonstrated by Dr. Lee and are now recognized by many informed researchers. Researchers are getting better at referring to synthetic progestins or natural progesterone and not using the terms interchangeably. Even conventional medicine is coming to a better understanding that women's health, hormone balance, nutrition, supplementation and exercise as an overall wholistic approach is directly related to a woman's emotional, mental and spiritual well-being.

As the Chief Medical Officer for Växa International, I continue to work with Cindy as we collaborate on new opportunities to guide women and all consumers with information and tools that will impact their lives to achieve optimal health. I can assure you that Cindy's research on women's health issues is based upon scientific principles of natural health and healing. The book offers information with empathy, caring and understanding, which comes directly from Cindy's unique ability to work in partnership with women to create the power of wholeness.

This book is the result of many years of research and listening to real women discuss real concerns, healthcare issues and challenges related to their struggles and successes in obtaining hormonal balance, wholeness and general well-being. Enjoy these invaluable "pearls" meant to enhance your daily life!

Stanley D. Headley, M.D., N.D.
Chief Medical Officer
VAXA International
Tampa, Florida

*"When health is absent, wisdom cannot reveal itself,
art cannot become manifest, strength cannot be exerted,
wealth is useless, and reason is powerless."*
—Herophilus, 300 B.C.

INTRODUCTION

EVERYBODY HAS A STORY TO TELL about how medicine has become like an assembly line; patients are being motored through a system, categorized as codes and procedures that equate to economics rather than as people getting their individual healthcare needs met.

The current healthcare delivery system has failed to provide us with healthcare solutions without introducing the risks and side effects of dangerous drugs or surgery.

As an example, when managing primary healthcare centers years ago, I challenged our practitioners to practice medicine without their prescription pads. They couldn't do it.

Many people, representing every socio-economic group, share stories about how they have been discarded by a system that no longer places their best interests first. They believe their healthcare providers are their advocates, yet the current healthcare delivery system is motivated more by profits and politics than patient advocacy.

Frustration abounds. Women, in particular, are searching for health solutions that will enable them to live vital lives and avoid chronic illnesses and diseases that are growing in epidemic proportions today. They want answers and are terribly confused about where to obtain good, honest information. Yet sometimes, despite the fact they are getting poor or no results from their personal healthcare providers, they continue to follow their advice. Could it be fear or a lack of confidence? Perhaps it is a little of both.

Many of my friends and colleagues placate me when I suggest they should learn about and be open to healthcare interventions that are safer and more effective. Hormone Replacement Therapy (HRT) is a good example.

For years I have been warning women about the dangers of HRT, warnings based on solid scientific evidence. In fact, some friends deliberately ignore me, even though they know my research background; they insist that their doctors would not steer them wrong. Fortunately or unfortunately, depending on how you look at it, I've been vindicated.

A colleague and friend of mine who is retiring from a 22-year career in the healthcare insurance business shared a conversation with me that she had with a male physician who had just been hired to replace her. During that conversation they talked about the ills that ail the healthcare delivery system today.

Having been entrenched in a 22-year career, she thought she had seen and heard it all. However, she was not prepared for what she was about to hear. He said, *"When patients get off their knees, physicians will come down from their pedestals."* This provocative comment illustrates one of the greatest health crises facing American women today.

In some inner circles, the medical letters 'M.D.' jokingly stand for 'Medical Deity'. Based upon the current conditions and attitudes of some professionals in our healthcare system today, this is not a joke.

The physician who replaced my friend made a point that was well taken. Many women, and men too, have relinquished their personal healthcare decisions and responsibilities to a profession that at one time was held in much higher esteem, a profession that has been hijacked by the pharmaceutical industry. Let me explain.

Pharmaceutical companies fund the majority of hospitals and medical school education in this country; these funds also pay for the majority of new drug studies and control the majority of updated medical information in medical journals physicians receive.

According to an article in the Wall Street Journal, June 13, 2003, the number of pharmaceutical representatives has tripled after a decade-long hiring spree in the 1990s to bring details about new medications and other treatments to physicians in their offices.

Drug company money is also the primary source of advertising dollars for TV and Magazines. Since Congress passed a law that allows drug companies to conduct "direct to consumer marketing," these sources have been a "golden goose" for the media.

The drug companies have stepped up their lobbying efforts to Congress, the U.S. and even foreign governments in order to further their economic interests. In 2003, The Pharmaceutical Research and Manufacturers of America (PhRMA) spent 23 per cent more than last year in support of their advertising efforts. Senator Richard J. Durbin (D-IL) and Senator Charles E. Schumer (D-NY) expressed their concern about the "death grip" this industry has on Congress and the antipathy felt by many toward the aggressive efforts to keep drug prices and drug company profits high.

U.S. Government regulators have launched an inquiry into whether a Canadian drug company has been paying kickbacks to U.S. doctors who prescribe a heart medication produced by the company. The inquiry, which is in its preliminary stages, is being conducted by the Health and Human Services Inspector General's Office and a U.S. Attorney's office. The company does not deny that they pay their physicians "compensation" which they feel generates physician survey data. And, of course, this "you take care of me and I'll take care of you" mentality is not new to the industry, but is not often made public.

Some physicians are not comfortable with the smothering tactics of the drug companies but it is difficult to walk away from such large sums of money. There is an over-emphasis on researching and funding patentable and profitable pharmaceuticals instead of encouraging equal amounts of research on natural vitamins and supplements.

*P*hysicians and other practitioners are forced to practice *"defensive medicine"* in order to decrease their risks of being sued, i.e., more testing is better. There is no advantage or incentive for practitioners to go outside the *"standard practice pattern"* even if it provides a better and safer outcome.

Punishment often awaits them in the form of being ostracized by peers, loss of referrals, lawsuits, a revoked medical license or being classified as a bonafide "quack".

Health Maintenance Organizations (HMO's) have monopolized the healthcare landscape during the past 20 years, forcing the entire healthcare industry to conform to their strategical tenets. Although their tenets are laudable and make good business sense, i.e. prevention, early detection and education, their practices are clearly the opposite.

The average office visit to an HMO practitioner is about five to eight minutes. This is more like a production line to get patients out faster, cut costs, avoid law suits and treat patient's symptoms rather than take time for a concise, clear examination. The typical medical treatment for almost any given healthcare condition or ailment consists of treating the symptom or killing the disease.

Nearly one in three doctors reports withholding information from patients about useful medical services that aren't covered by their health insurance companies and the number may be on the rise, according to the Institute for Ethics at the American Medical Association, commenting on a study reported in the journal, *Health Affairs*, 2003.

Is it any wonder why women are not getting the whole story or full disclosure of information when it comes to healthcare? In addition, women have spent the past few generations pursuing their dreams via the workforce in order to make viable and positive contributions, obtain self-efficacy, self-reliance, earning prestige and, in many cases, trying to make a living to feed and educate their families. This preoccupation has caused women to lose sight of their priorities and the many ways to influence their own health and healing, thus paving the way for others to make their personal healthcare decisions.

On the brighter side, there are many women in this country who are beginning to recognize the value of "good health", due to having suffered so long from many debilitating health conditions. Some women will not, and are not, depending on the broken healthcare delivery system to provide them the information they need to make more informed decisions. We need to encourage and support these women to become confident and courageous as they tackle their healthcare issues.

I formed **PRESERVION, Inc.**, a health information research, consultation and education company, born out of the need for women to obtain health information that has been researched and scientifically validated in order to help them make better and safer healthcare decisions for themselves and their families. Full disclosure of healthcare information screened from a health researcher/consumer advocate perspective enables healthcare consumers to decide which route of treatment and healing best suits them. This approach also removes the confusion of all the unfiltered information that is reported on a daily basis. It is that simple.

More women are looking for safer solutions that encourage healing versus treating symptoms. The treating symptom approach has failed women miserably. This should be no surprise. The next time you hear a drug advertisement on TV, listen carefully for the side effects of these treatments. It will go something like this: "Some side effects of the drugs may include liver damage, stroke, heart failure, migraine headaches, nausea, vomiting, black outs or other gastrointestinal upsets." And this is good, safe medicine? What's the upside?

Of course, many women turn to these drugs for immediate relief that in many cases works, at least in the short run. But the danger lies in that the use of many drugs prescribed to women for long term use not only begets the use of other drugs, but has no scientific history of being safe.

In September 2004, pharmaceutical giant Merck & Co. pulled its blockbuster arthritis drug, Vioxx, (considered to be a miraculous drug by many) from the market worldwide because new data from a clinical trial found an increased risk of heart attack and stroke. Yet, back in 2001, Vioxx was reported to have a "favorable cardiovascular safety profile." The FDA commented that given the rate of heart attacks and serious cardiovascular events reported from the use of this drug, it's incomprehensible that it took this long to pull it off the market.

This entire event of deception and withholding vital information from the public about a drug could be the last nail in the coffin for the pharmaceutical company, Merck. And don't be surprised when we begin to see more drugs being removed from the market for the same reasons. These egregious practices are starting to catch up to all the pharmaceutical manufacturers.

Later in this book, I will provide you with a historical perspective on the hormone replacement therapy (HRT) debacle, another example of what happens when decisions are based on bad scientific theory and unfettered enthusiasm.

All *good* science and research agrees and concludes that nothing functions by itself. The entire body is interrelated; body, mind and spirit. Our family, community, job, education, home, culture, religious beliefs and principles all work together and make us who we are. These functions also determine how we perceive *"health"* and how we make decisions about our health.

It's not a matter of discarding the randomized, double-blind, and controlled scientific studies considered the "gold standard", but of respecting and using other methodologies such as personal experiences, testimonials from patients, empirical data, clinical data and good, old-fashioned intuition and wisdom.

It is time to stop the dining and romancing of bizarre economics, self-interests, ugly politics, deceit, and manipulation of scientific data. It is time for all women to *get off their knees* and *stand up* and create profound changes in the way healthcare is delivered. Healthcare providers must place the best interests of their patients first.

Prevention is the key. Shifting from a disease-oriented model that treats symptoms to a model that supports the interrelated functions of the body and healing by identifying the underlying causes of dis-ease and illness, is the only way to create a *new model of medicine* that provides good, safe results and helps women heal.

Bright and intelligent women must regain control of their own health and healthcare and help to re-educate their physicians and other healthcare practitioners. Do not dismiss answers or suggestions you get because they seem silly, contrary or unconventional to what you have been taught to believe. If the conventional answers were satisfactory, you would not have had to ask the questions in the first place.

Women's healthcare conditions and diseases are growing in

epidemic proportions. You do not need to be a statistic of this growing phenomenon. Women will learn that drugs and surgery should be left as an absolute last resort — not as a first choice. They will also gain a clear understanding that they are not a diseased species, but rather a gifted species that has the ability of bringing new life into this world. With this gift comes physiological, emotional and biological changes that need a little assistance throughout a lifetime.

My purpose for writing this book is to share my passion, scientific research, professional experiences and knowledge of 25 years in order to infuse a renewed enthusiasm and desire in women to learn how to stay healthy and how to create and manage a personal health plan to live better longer. Facts and opinions are presented in the spirit of challenging the medical mainstream's arguments versus attacking anyone's personal character.

I would like to believe that what I write in this book will go beyond these pages and touch people in a way that will inspire them to learn how to obtain and maintain optimal health. And I hope and pray that my writings will contribute to someone's healthy living and greatness that will inspire others.

You are about to embark on a new journey that will introduce you to the true concepts of prevention, healing, healthy living and choices.

"When you sell a woman a book you don't just sell her
paper, ink and glue, you sell her a whole new life!
There's heaven and earth in a real book. The real purpose
of books is to inspire the mind to do its own thinking!"
—Christopher Morely

1

A TIME FOR CHANGE

A LARGE CONSTITUENCY OF WOMEN have already decided
to find their own answers. They are troubled by the ineffec-
tiveness of their medical treatment and the side effects of their
drugs. They do not necessarily doubt the sincerity and intelli-
gence of their physicians. However, they are concerned by their
healthcare providers' apparent indifference to the toxic side
effects that remain after prescribed medications are used and by
the rate at which prescriptions are written.

Women are so hungry for good information that they are
attending seminars, reading books, doing research and talking
amongst themselves to gain feedback and comfort in sharing
what has become a common threat to their well-being.

Women must work toward becoming more informed and
confident, sorting out truths from myths and include intuition
in making personal healthcare decisions. Women gaining information will create a *"new medicine"* that will focus on the whole
body. This *"new medicine"* will:

- insist that prevention and treatment are equally important to overall wellness.

- embrace the importance of self-responsibility, good nutrition, supplements, exercise, self-awareness, relaxation, spirituality and prayer.
- teach women that they can heal themselves without drugs and surgery and without scorn from uninformed healthcare professionals.
- create *"health"*.

There is good reasoning behind this approach. Despite popular opinion, United States citizens do *not* have the best health in the world. A commentary in the July 26, 2000 issue of *Journal of the American Medical Association* asks, "Is healthcare in the U.S. really the best in the world?" It cites a report of the overall health performance data of 16 advanced nations. Japan ranks first. The U.S. ranks 12th out of the 16 developed nations.

In the U.S. we spend $5,000 per person per year on healthcare, almost double that of Switzerland, the next most expensive country. There is obviously a lack of any clear connection between increased spending and better health. The U.S. spends in excess of 95 percent of its healthcare dollars on curative strategies and less than 5 percent on prevention.

J. M. McGinniss and W.H. Foege's paper, *"Actual Causes of Death,"* yields the inescapable inference that poor health and most modern day illnesses are directly related to lifestyle behaviors and can be avoided through a preventive approach.

Another study conducted by the Rand Corporation, a respected, nonpartisan research firm, reported that Americans receive the correct healthcare treatment less than 60 percent of the time, resulting in unnecessary pain, expense and death. *"It is somewhat outrageous that we spend $1.4 trillion on healthcare and get it right only half the time,"* says Elizabeth McGlynn, the lead author of the study.

Many consumers are without insurance and suffer from some of the most devastating contraindications from state-of-the-art pharmaceutical drugs. Due to medical errors, our healthcare system is the number one cause of death compared to other nations. These include unnecessary surgeries, medication errors in hospitals, other errors and infection rates in hospitals, adverse effects of prescribed medications and iatrogenic (due to treatments by physicians) causes.

Unlike natural approaches to health and healing that have stood the test of time, our modern medical model is constantly reversing opinions. Consider what author/surgeon Sherwin B. Nuland notes:

- Is radical mastectomy the best treatment for breast cancer?
- Is drinking coffee associated with an increased risk of pancreatic malignancy?
- Should every ruptured spleen be removed?
- Is a low-fiber diet the best treatment for chronic diverticulitis?
- Is acid production by the stomach the key factor in peptic ulcer?
- Should every man, or nearly all men, with prostate cancer have surgery?
- Are most cases of impotence psychosomatic?

The answer to every one of these questions was once "Yes" and is now "No."

The healthier we are as people, the better off we, as a nation, will be. It is imperative that healthcare decisions are made by you, the consumer, not the politicians, bureaucrats or gatekeepers. You must learn how to avoid the medical maze and take charge. I've provided a practical approach.

First Steps…How to Relate to Your Doctor

Partnering with your healthcare practitioner is good medicine. Patients who ask questions, do a little research and get 2nd and 3rd opinions, motivate their practitioners — informed practitioners, that is — to give them more information because these patients are perceived as being personally involved and intelligent.

The quality of healthcare you receive depends largely on your ability to communicate with your healthcare practitioner.

If your healthcare practitioner is not meeting your needs, or is unwilling to talk to you and answer your questions, please, find one who will. There are many good practitioners who are highly dedicated to their profession and are committed to working with you.

How to Choose a Practitioner

This is not always an easy task, particularly when you are looking for someone to work with in providing answers to this *"new medicine"*. A good starting point begins with exploring the following issues:

- Ask a friend or family member. Ask friends who share your philosophy on health and prevention for a recommendation. Your friends and family know you and if they use practitioners who share your philosophy they will be a good source to determine whether your philosophies and personalities will be compatible.
- Contact an accredited hospital. Inquire about their commitment to health and prevention and whether or not they are open to integrative healthcare practices. If they are, ask to speak to practitioners who have a history of practicing medicine that supports health and healing.

- Contact a local healthcare practitioner who has developed a good reputation. Make an appointment to meet with him/her. Most practitioners will be willing to meet you for a consultation at no cost to determine whether you are a good match. This is the time to ask about their medical achievements, to make sure you feel comfortable with this person and that they share your philosophy about health.
- Search the internet. There are multiple websites that will list practitioners and their biographies, where they attended school, their training, experience and level of expertise in their specialty.
- Contact The American Holistic Association. They have compiled a list of practitioners who work in partnership with their patients, and encourage a wholistic approach to wellness. http://ahha.org/ahre.htm
- Check with medical associations affiliated with different specialties.

WHAT TO EXPECT FROM A GOOD PRACTITIONER

Does he/she:
- listen to you?
- explain his/her findings?
- answer your questions?
- remain open to your suggestions?
- carefully examine you?
- take time with you?
- keep up with the latest scientific literature?
- make you feel comfortable?
- have an office staff that is attentive and knowledgeable?
- look at you wholistically rather than as a symptom or pain?

Getting the Most out of your Office Visit

- Prepare a list of questions prior to your visit.
- Write down responses from your healthcare practitioner or use a tape recorder.
- Never assume that a hospital or a nurse or a doctor's office will do any coordinating of the big picture. Patients with complicated health challenges need an advocate to help them.
- Don't hesitate to bring a friend to be a second set of ears.
- Do research on your illness/condition if possible.
- Ask questions. Always ask why.
- Bring medical records or results from previous tests administered. Inform your healthcare practitioner about any sensitivity you have to medications/herbs/supplements.
- Inform your healthcare practitioner about any medications/herbs/supplements and the doses you are currently taking.
- Know your medical history, including past illnesses and hospitalizations.

Testing

If your doctor suggests a test of any kind, ask him to be specific about foods, medications or other factors that might affect the results. For instance, a blood test to determine cholesterol levels requires nine to 12 hours of fasting before the blood is drawn. Without the fast, levels could easily be high enough to prompt many doctors to prescribe a statin drug.

Remember, medicine is an *ART.*

A... Ask questions.

R... Research

T... Take control of your health care.

WHAT TO ASK ABOUT PRESCRIPTION DRUGS

- What problem are these drugs trying to solve?
- Is it a life or death situation?
- By solving this problem, what other problems have I created?
- Does the benefit outweigh the risk?
- Who benefits most from this drug?
- Is there an alternative that is safer?
- How long do I need to take this drug before I can expect a positive impact? How long must I be on the drug?
- When will I be retested to evaluate whether or not I can stop using the drug?

WHAT TO ASK ABOUT SURGERY

- How will I benefit from this surgery?
- How will the surgery improve my quality of life and/or my chances of survival?
- What are the risks/benefits of having this surgery? What can happen if I do not have the surgery?
- What are the alternatives to this surgery?
- What percentage of these types of surgeries are successful? Can we take a "wait and watch" approach to avoid this surgery?

Take this list along with you every time you visit a health-care practitioner. By expressing yourself and taking charge, you make it clear that you take yourself and your health seriously and expect others to do so.

A large constituency of women, along with some men, are creating the demand for this transformation of "*new medicine*." This is a very exciting time and great things are happening for those who take responsibility for their own health. The foundation of this greatness lies in education. The time for change is now.

"When you eventually see through the veil to how things really are, you will keep saying again and again, this is certainly not like we thought it was!"
—*Mevlana Jalaluddin Rumi*

2

HORMONE REPLACEMENT THERAPY (HRT)...TRUTHS VERSUS HALF-TRUTHS

REMEMBER WHEN YOU DID *NOT* GO to the doctor for a headache, sore throat, or cold and got better in seven days anyway? Do you remember when you went to your family doctor and he sat down with genuine interest to discuss why you came to see him? Do you remember when the doctor told you to go home, drink a little ginger ale, eat some dry toast and get a little rest and call him in the morning? That's all changed now. The practice of medicine has changed forever and so must you!

THE JOURNALS AND HEADLINES READ:

- Women's Health Initiative (WHI) study halted due to significant health risks for women taking Estrogen-Progestin, *National Institute of Health (NIH)* July, 2002
- Menopausal Hormone Replacement and Risk of Ovarian Cancer, *Journal of the American Medical Association JAMA*, July 17, 2002
- Trial of Hormone Replacement Therapy to prevent

coronary heart disease halted early because of increased harm, *Lancet,* July 13, 2002

- Estrogen Put on Federal Government's List of Carcinogens, *Washington Post,* December, 2002
- Hormone Pills Don't Help Most Women, Study Says, *Nation/World,* March 18, 2003
- A New Danger for Women on Hormones: Latest Study Finds Sharp Increase in Dementia for Prempro Users-few reasons to continue therapy, *Wall Street Journal,* May 28, 2003
- New Risk in Taking Prempro: Murky Mammograms, *Wall Street Journal,* June 25, 2003
- Study Reveals Hormone Therapy Risk: Heart Attack Chance Doubles for Women, *Nation/World,* August 7, 2003
- Breast Cancer Risk from Hormone Therapy Reaffirmed, *Tampa Tribune,* August 8, 2003
- Study Casts New Doubt on Hormones: Estrogen-Progestin may raise cancer risk, *Associated Press,* 2003
- Study Shows Hormone Link to Dementia, *New York Times,* 2003
- Hormone Therapy Debate Grows, *Wall Street Journal,* October, 2003

There is strong, conclusive evidence that states clearly that hormone replacement therapy (HRT) is *no* longer the drug of choice for pre-menopause or menopausal symptoms, coronary heart disease, dementia or osteoporosis.

SUMMARY OF FINDINGS:
WOMEN'S HEALTH INITIATIVE (WHI) 2002

March 2002   Hormone replacement therapy fails to improve older women's memory, sleeping or mental outlook, as many had assumed.

May 2002   Those who took estrogen/progestin an average of more than four years face double the risk of Alzheimer's or other forms of dementia.

June 2002   Breast cancer linked to estrogen-progestin pills may be fast-growing and hard to detect.

July 2002   Government-backed Women's Health Initiative (WHI) study of 16,608 women is halted because researchers discover significant health risks for women taking estrogen-progestin pills. Risk of heart disease is 29 percent higher than expected and breast cancer risk increases by 26 percent.

August 2002   The risk of heart attacks during the first year on the pills is nearly double the expected rate. Risk is also higher than expected for those with elevated levels of bad cholesterol.

While the so-called "experts" on women's health are reassuring women that there are only minor, unpleasant side-effects, Dr. Lynette J. Dumble, Senior Research Fellow at the University of Melbourne's Department of Surgery at the Royal Melbourne Hospital, believes that the sole basis of HRT is to create a commercial market that is highly profitable for the pharmaceutical companies and doctors. The findings in this study were far from "minor."

Yet despite all the documented evidence, many physicians, institutions and medical authorities in this country continue to prescribe and encourage the use of synthetic HRT and, at the same time, assure women that the risks are very low.

There is simply no logic to this behavior; HRT has been pervasively injected into our culture and is killing us slowly. Many other false messages about what cures women's health conditions are circulating as well.

To add insult to injury, using a dangerous drug treatment that significantly increases the risk of death and disability as a balm for discomfort is insidious and borders on criminal. This is like playing a game of Russian Roulette. You just don't know when or if you will become a statistic.

Emory University and the National Cancer Society published a report on an eight-year study of over 240,000 women, which found that the women who were on estrogen alone had a 72 percent higher risk of ovarian cancer.

In 1997, a study published in the *Lancet* concluded that HRT increased the risk of breast cancer with each year of use. The *Medical Tribune* reported that after ten years of use, Estrogen Replacement Therapy (ERT) increased a woman's risk of dying from breast cancer by 43 percent. How is it that we had to wait so long for this study to end? HRT and ERT should have never been prescribed in the first place because earlier studies had indicated risks.

*J*erilynn Prior, MD, a world authority in endocrinology, says that describing menopause as an "estrogen deficiency disease" is the same as describing a headache as an "aspirin deficiency disease." She calls this type of thinking "backwards science." Illnesses cannot be categorized by which drugs they are missing. That would assume that drugs cure illnesses, which is rarely the case, especially when referring to HRT. Besides, menopause is not an illness and does not require drugs.

The British Medical Journal (BMJ) devoted several articles to how drug companies profit from medicalizing the everyday trials and tribulations of life. According to some of the authors, the drug-company strategy is relatively simple: Create anxiety about possible health problems in relatively healthy people so that they ask their physicians for treatment. This is disease mongering. Some of the BMJ authors say that the emphasis on drug treatment takes attention away from modestly effective non-pharmaceutical strategies, such as dietary supplementation with calcium and vitamin D, smoking cessation and weight-bearing exercise. No truer words have been spoken.

A LITTLE HISTORY

Ayerst Pharmaceutical Company, known as Wyeth Ayerst today, was the first maker of conjugated estrogen (a combination of several estrogens) better known as PREMARIN, or estrogen replacement therapy (ERT), made from pregnant mare's urine, thus the name, PRE-MAR-IN. The idea of prescribing a product of horse's urine for human consumption is, in itself, sufficient cause for questioning its efficacy.

From 1965 to the early 1970s, everything appeared to be going along well until something ugly began happening. Women began developing uterine cancer (an overgrowth of the lining of the uterus from the horse estrogen) at a rate four to eight times greater than those *not* taking Premarin. When this news reached the public, women became very concerned and the use of the "magic pill" dropped precipitously.

Rather than pulling this drug off the market, the company retooled. They realized the financial impact this had on them and they quickly concluded with *minimal* research conducted by the Medical College of Georgia and the Goldwater Memorial Hospital in New York City that women on a treatment of synthetic progestin (natural progesterone chemically altered into a patentable drug) plus estrogen had a lower incidence of uterine cancer than those not taking the hormones.

Studies have proven that this new drug had life threatening risks like breast cancer, heart disease, and Alzheimer's disease. Nonetheless, this information was ignored. At that time, ERT was renamed hormone replacement therapy (HRT) by combining the two drugs and remarketed as PremPro. Thus began the enthusiastic promotion of a new drug with very little science to support its safety and efficacy long term.

The phase of menopause, which *is natural* in a woman's life, had been fabricated into a diseased state. Unfortunately, pregnancy which is natural too, has also been classified as a disease state; another painful irony.

Women are not sick nor are they unhealthy due to menopause. Some women experience debilitating symptoms during the transition of moving from a period of fertility to non-fertility. This does not mean that drugs are the answer, even though this country is driven by the mindset that modern technology and the pharmaceutical industry have the answers to correct every known health problem.

Louise knew better. She contacted me after becoming terribly frustrated with her doctor during an office visit. At the age of 62, she had lost her desire for sexual relations with her husband because of vaginal dryness that caused her pain during intercourse. She was feeling anxious about the situation and was not sleeping well. Unlike many women, her transition during menopause was uneventful in that she hardly experienced any negative effects and did not require any type of hormone treatment or medications.

When her physician prescribed HRT and Prozac to help her ease these symptoms, she was shocked. She was not interested in any type of HRT due to the health risks reported in many studies, and she was offended that her doctor suggested an antidepressant drug to calm her and help her sleep. Intuitively, she did not feel comfortable about this recommendation.

I agreed with Louise. I suggested the use of vitamin E oil during intercourse and the use of a little natural progesterone crème applied to the skin daily for three weeks each month to benefit the vaginal tissue. This course of action is often recommended in many scientific journals and books.

Louise was very encouraged by this recommendation and expressed a sigh of relief in that these natural approaches, if successful, would not put her at risk. I followed up with Louise one month later to learn that she was feeling much better, sleeping better and enjoying sexual relations with her husband once again. Her feelings of anxiousness completely diminished and she was thankful that she did not concede to the recommendations of her physician. I suggested she continue this regime for about three to four months to encourage her body to retain balance, and to continue the vitamin E oil indefinitely. I also encouraged her to share these results with her doctor. Often times, it is a simple, non-medical approach that can improve some of the most common health issues.

In the 1970s, Consumer Reports documented our grotesque overuse of prescription and over-the-counter drugs. Americans use five to seven billion of the tranquilizers Valium and Librium, and 20,000 tons or 225 aspirin per adult per year. Imagine the dependency consumers have placed on prescription and over-the-counter drugs today!

Something is terribly wrong with this ideology. Children are prescribed drugs that in the past were only used for adults; it's getting more difficult to find someone in their 40s who isn't taking a synthetic hormone, an anti-cholesterol drug, blood pressure medication or an antidepressant; and pediatric physicians are now recommending cholesterol screening for children as young as two.

Antidepressant use among young Americans has been growing 10 percent a year. Only just recently has the FDA confirmed that the risks of their use outweigh their benefits. Yet back in 2003, warnings were being sent to doctors about the possible risks to children of a newer generation of antidepressant drugs. Is there a movement in this country by the current bio-medical model to "medicalize" everyday life beginning with our children?

There is the prevailing question that haunts many of us regarding the use of powerful drugs. Some women are beginning to ask why doctor's attitudes and judgments are condescending and why there is such a rush to prescribe drugs and perform surgeries. Could the answer be that women's health and welfare is secondary to their own convenience and economic gain? Is our health being traded on Wall Street where the price determines which disease should be considered and which should be ignored?

The history and science behind the devastating effects of HRT are riveting. Many doctors still tell women not to worry and that the use of HRT is safe. Adding more fuel to the fire was an article written in the Wall Street Journal in which physicians subscribe to the notion that the science is flawed in the Women's Health Initiative (WHI) study that was halted in 2003 (three years earlier than expected) due to a greater risk of invasive breast cancer, heart disease and strokes among women using PREMPRO (Premarin plus Provera).

Representatives from Harvard Medical School, Brigham and Women's Hospital, Stanford University and other practicing physicians believe that the Women's Health Initiative study went a bit overboard. As critics, they contest that the study was about older women and that there is no reason that young women should feel threatened or at risk when using synthetic hormones. This is an interesting comment since young women age to become older women. And we know that lifestyle choices made early in life directly affect us as we age and determine the outcome of our health status later in life.

This thinking has become quite polarizing in medical circles, as it should be. If the research used to study these women is supposedly the gold standard, then, the outcome should be as good as gold, right? Again, it looks more like a drug looking for a disease. This scenario is what confuses women as they attempt to relieve their symptoms.

By seeking symptom-only relief, the desire or need to look for the cause falls by the wayside. Profits prevail over good science again and the controversy continues.

AN OFFICE VISIT

Mary went to her gynecologist for her annual visit and was told to stop using natural progesterone cream due to the WHI study showing the dangerous effects of progestin and estrogen in combination. Her doctor said that natural progesterone had the same effect of increasing the risk of breast cancer as did progestin. Nothing is further from the truth.

Sad to say, this is the proverbial response by many practicing physicians. Much of this is due to a lack of knowledge, information shared within inner circles, and articles written in conventional medical journals. Detailed pharmaceutical representatives are feeding physicians just enough information to sell their drugs and these practitioners are on the defense when approached by a more informed patient.

Natural versus Synthetic Hormones

Natural progesterone (a bio-identical hormone) replicates the body's own progesterone that is made by the adrenal glands or by the ovaries as a consequence of ovulation. Thus, it is called *natural.* The synthetic hormones, Provera (medroxyprogesterone acetate) and Premarin (conjugated estrogen) have been molecularly altered and differ in molecular configuration from hormones made by the body.

NATURAL PROGESTERONE IN COMPARISON TO PROGESTINS

Natural Progesterone	Synthetic Progestins
Protects against ovarian cancer	Increases sodium and water in body cells
Protects against endometrial cancer	Causes loss of mineral electrolytes from cells
Protects against breast cancer	Causes intracellular edema
Normalizes libido	Causes depression
Causes less hirsutism, regrowth of hair	Increases birth defect risks
Improves lipid profile	Causes facial hirsutism, loss of scalp hair
Improves new bone formation	Causes embolism risk
Decreases risk of coronary vasospasm	Decreases glucose tolerance
Facilitates thyroid hormone action	Causes allergy reactions
Effective in treating PMS	Increases risk of cholestatic jaundice
Necessary for successful pregnancy	Causes acne and skin rashes
Restores normal sleep patterns	Increases risk of coronary vasospasm
Is a precursor of other steroid hormones	Prevents fertilized ovum from occurring

Chart A - Used with permission from *What Your Doctor May Not Tell You About Premenopause,* John R.Lee, M.D., 1999.

Therefore, hormones that are *not* bio-identical do *not* provide the same physiological activity as the ones they are intended to replace. This is plain and simple physiology 101, yet medical institutions and the like have chosen to ignore this information. Medical professionals who espouse this simple physiologic concept are considered quacks, are often ridiculed and accused of having no credibility. Keep in mind, however, that only when hormones are synthesized, (changing molecular structure), can they be patentable and sold for billions of dollars. The pharmaceutical companies have taken perfectly normal plants and have changed the molecular structure in order to turn profits! Is the picture getting clearer?

The history of the production of synthetic drugs shows that when a so-called active ingredient is separated from the whole plant, a substance not known to nature is created and almost always causes harmful side effects. Therefore, plant medicines are almost always safer when used properly in their natural form. Mother Nature does know best!

There is little incentive to research natural progesterone or any other natural hormones because they cannot be patented. Secondly, synthetic hormones are much more potent and are always prescribed in excessively high dosages (and the same amount to every woman). This prescribing practice is due to the fact that the majority of the substance breaks down through the liver and digestive process before it can be semi-effective. The reason why the patches and topical crèmes are so potent is because the skin as an organ is extremely permeable.

NOT BY HORMONES ALONE

A reporter interviewed Dr. Margery Glass, professor of Clinical Obstetrics and Gynecology at the University of Cincinnati, College of Medicine. Dr. Glass stated that natural (bio-identical hormones) and synthetic hormones affect the body in the same manner. I disagree. The history of synthetic hormones is very clear, as shown in the research provided in this book.

Often overlooked is basic physiology that takes a back seat to more exciting research such as the production of new drugs, DNA testing, treating disease, the human genome, and human cloning or any other potential research that may generate big dollars.

Many articles and even scientific journals will use the term "progestin" and "progesterone" interchangeably, as though they were one and the same. These two terms refer to two entirely different chemistries.

Progestin is invented (synthetic); therefore, it does not occur in nature. It has been molecularly altered; therefore, the body finds it very difficult to metabolize and excrete. As a result of this alteration, it cannot be used as a precursor to other hormones and causes serious side effects.

Progesterone, on the other hand, is a precursor of other hormones such as estrogen, testosterone, and corticosteroids. It is made from the sterol pregnenolone, which in turn is made from cholesterol. It is metabolized by the body, passes through the liver and then excreted. Something so simple and clearly detailed in chemistry should not be misunderstood. Yet, I sense sometimes that there is a deliberate attempt to confuse consumers.

This is how and why many of our institutions and the physicians who represent them are losing credibility. There are a growing number of women who are learning how to take charge of their own health, regardless of what physicians and medical institutions say. Women are no longer buying their blather. Why should they? The evidence is crystal clear.

Another study, conducted in Sweden, involved over 23,000 women. Overall it was noted that there was a 10 percent increase in the relative risk of breast cancer for 23,334 women for whom estrogens were prescribed to alleviate symptoms of menopause.

ANOTHER UNFORTUNATE TREND

There is also a growing trend of disdain for natural and safe products in the medical world, now that some women are taking charge. How can anyone criticize the use of natural remedies such as epsons salts (magnesium sulfate), milk of magnesia and other natural and safe products that have been effective throughout the years prior to the pharmaceutical industry medicalizing simple ailments? Our medical model has lost its way, having been hijacked by the pharmaceutical giants.

Nature has always provided. Throughout the ages, plants have been used for medicinal purposes. Animals will eat grass and other greens when they have a need for more chlorophyll (green pigment in plants) or need a laxative. Chlorophyll helps to cleanse the bowels and prevent constipation. Saw palmetto, kava kava, garlic, and ginko biloba, to name a few, have been used for centuries to address several types of maladies and conditions. Because plants are just like humans at the molecular level, it makes sense that the body would respond favorably and without the risks posed by pharmacological agents. Even though it has hundreds of years of experience, the medical community continues to drive fear into consumers about the use of natural products.

There is too much criticism and hostility coming from the mouths of our medical establishment. Their comments may reflect their personal fears after seeing that what they have been taught is not all good science and is losing credibility. Jealousy, resentment, the *NIH* syndrome (not invented here) or just good old-fashioned arrogance is folded into the attitude and practices of too many. Regardless of the intent, these words sting and stay in the minds of patients for a lifetime.

THE MILLION WOMEN STUDY

Not only did results of the WHI study shatter what was conceived and perceived as *fact*, but on the heels of this information were the results of another study conducted across the Atlantic.

The *Lancet* reported on the Million Women Study (MWS) conducted in the United Kingdom. The purpose of the study was to measure the impact HRT had on women's health issues and the risk of developing breast cancer. The study concluded that women who used HRT had a substantially greater risk of breast cancer and a greater risk of dying from it.

The MWS is the largest study of its kind and the first one to report an increase in risk of death from breast cancer for those using HRT compared with women who never used it. The researchers also found that all combinations of synthetic hormones, including progestin and estrogen together, or estrogen alone, increased the risk of breast cancer.

The use of HRT by women ages 50-64 in the United Kingdom over the past ten years has resulted in an estimated 20,000 extra breast cancers, 15,000 of which are associated with estrogen and progestin combination. The longer women took HRT, the greater their risk of breast cancer. This should be no surprise based on research on Chart A, on page 42, that shows the contraindications of these synthetic hormones.

Why didn't our news media make this headline news? Whether the combination of hormones listed in this study was taken orally or topically, the evidence validated the increased risk of breast cancer.

The good news extrapolated from the study showed that the risk of breast cancer declined gradually after women stopped using these hormones; and within five years of quitting their use, they had the same risk as women who had never used them.

HAVEN'T THEY LEARNED YET?

Estrasorb, the first topical estrogen therapy, has been approved by the Food and Drug Administration (FDA) to treat moderate to severe vasomotor (hot flashes). The advantage, supposedly, is that it is a lotion women love, and it is easy to apply to the skin.

What is so disturbing about this statement is that published data consistently shows synthetic estrogen to be carcinogenic and causes multiple side effects regardless of how it is used or in what combination. This is why it is imperative to do your research regardless of what conventional institutions espouse.

Why are drug companies and physicians still trying to promote the use of a dangerous drug that has been studied thoroughly? Why is there even an argument about this treatment? Money, energy and time should and could be placed into researching natural and safer solutions that "do no harm" to women.

*I*t is no surprise that drug companies are driven by profits and have used their power to influence many areas of medicine. Unfortunately, their influence has resulted in many biased studies, which mislead the public.

A phase III randomized, controlled, double blind trial was conducted by none other than the maker of this crème, NOVAVAX. This is like the fox guarding the henhouse. How was this approved by the FDA?

Dr. Benjamin Rush, personal physician to George Washington stated, "*Unless we put medical freedom into the constitution, the time will come when medicine will organize into an underground dictatorship...To restrict the art of healing to one class of men and deny equal privileges to others will constitute the Bastille of medical science. All such laws are un-American and despotic and have no place in a republic...The constitution of this republic should make special privilege for medical freedom as well as religious freedom.*" Have we learned anything yet?

The WHI study and the MWS concluded that HRT (estrogen and progestin in combination as well as estrogen alone) is dangerous. This example is not intended to single out a particular doctor, but to demonstrate how misinformation circulates into the medical circles and how medical institutions and physicians can perpetuate such misinformation even after it has been disproved.

ADVERTISING AND ITS IMPACT ON WOMEN

When a practicing physician reads this type of research in medical journals or hears about it from colleagues, patterns in the practice of medicine begin to emerge. Then come the documentaries, the announcements on the radio, the newspaper articles, the nightly news, and the billboards on the buses, trains and in subways.

This misguided information surrounds us constantly and the images influence our thinking and decision making. So, if your friend is using HRT and tells you her doctor said it was safe, you conclude that it is safe for you also.

From the example of the physician who determined that natural progesterone is the same as synthetic progestin, due to the half truths presented in journals, we can see how misinformation circulates rapidly.

St. James, the apostle, gave an example of a ship's rudder and likened it to the tongue of humans when communicating. Although they are both small, they are very powerful in nature and guide with great boasts. Communicating information that is incorrect can set a course for a lifetime that is very difficult to undo. The case of hormone replacement therapy has been set boastfully, and has been on a destructive course for too long.

Professional experiences, observations, research and personal stories from clients lead me to believe that our medical model is dehumanizing women under the guise of offering a safer, better and more convenient way of living. Communicating honest medical information seems to have gotten lost in the human appetite for greed, power and control. Women have been treated very shabbily by being given partial disclosure of health-care information. As a result of this attitude, HRT over the past few years has pitted many professionals against one another and against their patients, too.

FIGHTING TILL THE END

Even after all the negative study results, it looks like the use of HRT is not going down without a fight. In Canada, the OB/GYN's are still promoting the use of this dangerous drug, even after a recent statement announced by the Canadian Cancer

Society advised women *not to* take HRT. Period!

Doctors contend that it is safe for a limited amount of time. They say it does not become dangerous until the five-year mark, and their statistics show that most women in Canada take HRT for only three years.

All informed women and physicians should gather together and form a rebuttal to the type of irresponsibility described above. The science says it is *not* safe, yet they choose to ignore it. Women must challenge this mindset in order to avoid harm's way. It is no wonder women are beginning to take health matters into their own hands.

CAROL'S STORY

Carol ended up in a shouting match with her doctor over HRT. She wanted his help with natural, bio-identical hormone replacement, but like the physicians in Canada, he tried to convince her that a little "Prempro" wouldn't hurt her. When she refused his recommendations and countered them by citing all the studies, he literally yelled at her. Apparently, this physician is not used to a more informed patient making personal decisions about her own healthcare. Trying to reform and educate physicians like this is like trying to roast snowballs.

This type of behavior is appalling and all too common. One would think that after a major study had been halted due to the dangers, medical professionals would be asking, "What do we do now?" Rather, we are seeing increased bickering and anger between professionals and patients. No one wins with this type of attitude.

ROGER

"My wife is so angry at her doctor that she can barely bring herself to see him again." For years the doctor told her to take Premarin and Provera. When reports began to reach the public that there might be a problem with an increase of breast cancer, she asked him about this risk. He repeatedly reassured her that there was nothing to worry about. "Hormones are so safe," he claimed, that his own wife was taking them.

Have we all heard this before? A patient will ask a doctor what he or she would do if it were their mother or sister, and if they reply in the affirmative, then it is perceived to be relevant and safe for the patient. This is not particularly unreasonable thinking; however, when the family members of these physicians begin to be diagnosed with breast cancer, uterine cancer or other female problems, they consider it the norm because the majority of women have the same outcomes! They think nothing of this. This is unreasonable!

TEAM WORK

Physicians and women should be working together as a team to come up with solutions. Physicians need to listen to their patients and become more cognizant of where they are getting their medical information, regardless of community practices by their colleagues.

There is ample evidence that the original research on hormones was inadequate, sloppy and driven by profits over safety and scientific validity. What are the current medical institutions, authorities and researchers doing to assure women that the information being communicated today is valid? What are they doing to restore the confidence that most women once had in them? Women, BEWARE!!!

A lesson all women can and should take away from this ordeal is that it is most important to find a physician or healthcare practitioner who can be trusted. Engage in dialogue and begin discussions before any medical decision is made. The use of synthetic hormones is dangerous at best. Women should consider using natural hormones (bio-identical) if there is a clinical need. It's not that hormones are bad. They are necessary for the body's organs to work in concert with one another. Balance, or homeostatis, is the key. When women's hormones are in balance, their bodies will function beautifully.

By now, we should all understand why women should *never* use synthetic hormones—not even for a short time. Why take the risk? We know that, from here on in, we do *not* want to continue down this treacherous path of deceit, self-serving propensities and shoddy science. Women must take personal responsibility and work in partnership with one another, their physicians and other professional health advocates who have their best interests at heart.

The next time your doctor suggests the use of any synthetic hormones, refer him/her to this book or books on similar topics. If he/she is not interested, I suggest you find another doctor.

One last thing to keep in mind is that clinical medicine, which we have been discussing, is an imperfect science, is an experiment and is unpredictable. In fact, medicine is more of an art because we, as humans, are *not* machines. With that said, we as individuals require an artful approach. It is science, not medicine that has helped us understand more about the natural processes of our bodies and how they work. And if science and the facts determined health policy in this country, prevention and health would be the foundation of healthcare practices, instead of emergency medicine, treatment and drugs.

These facts should help women discern truth from fiction. We now know that synthetic hormone replacement therapy is risky and should be avoided.

I like what Max Planck, renowned Nobel Prize winner of Physics in 1918, says about the truth and science:

"A new scientific truth does not triumph by convincing its opponents and making them see the light, but rather because its opponents eventually die, and a new generation grows up that is familiar with it."

"The price of greatness is responsibility.
So take that responsibility for your life,
and great things will happen."
—Winston Churchill

3

BALANCING HORMONES...
A SAFER AND GENTLER APPROACH

NEWS ABOUT THE OUTCOMES of the Women's Health Initiative and the Million Women Study have now been placed in the hands of women this past year and as a result, the use of Premarin and Prempro has dropped dramatically.

It was reported by a prescription tracker in Atlanta in 2003, after the results were made public about the WHI study, that Premarin usage dropped to 2.7 million prescriptions from 5.6 million and Prempro usage dropped from 3.4 million prescriptions to 1.2 million. Thank goodness. With more information being reported daily on the risks of synthetic hormones, I suspect the numbers will continue falling.

Informed women are searching for and using safer solutions to alleviate symptoms during menopause, a transitional stage in life that occurs in three phases:

- perimenopause, a transitional period,
- menopause, the end of perimenopause and the start of a new era, and
- post-menopause, menstruation has completely ceased.

During this entire transitional period, many women are struggling to deal with symptoms that affect their daily lives, symptoms that result from biological, emotional, physical and hormonal changes. These changes occur because the ovaries no longer produce eggs or the physiological amounts of estrogen and progesterone that they produced at a younger age.

Many women in their early to mid thirties begin to experience erratic menstrual cycles, infertility, uterine fibroids, painful breasts, premenstrual syndrome (PMS), mood swings, weight gain, depression, migraine headaches, and many other symptoms. All of these symptoms occur due to several factors such as: the use of HRT, hormone imbalances or estrogen dominance (a term coined by Dr. John R. Lee). Estrogen dominance is due to the exposure of excessive estrogen in many forms plus not enough progesterone due to hysterectomy, poor diet, lack of exercise, and lack of proper nutritional supplements.

The good news is that there are many different approaches a woman can pursue to overcome the symptoms that cause discomfort and to help put her body on a healing path during menopause. Linda Page, N.D., Ph.D. says it beautifully. *"Menopause is actually nature's way of protecting women from breast and uterine cancer by rebalancing hormone production - a process that no one should try to defeat with pharmaceuticals."*

If you are currently using synthetic hormones, please do not stop taking them abruptly. Work with a healthcare professional who will help you slowly wean yourself from them. This will help to ease the many symptoms that may occur while in this transition. At the same time, incorporate the following lifestyle behaviors to assist you in the healing process.

LET THE HEALING BEGIN WITH SUPPLEMENTS

Take a good multivitamin that includes minerals, amino acids and essential fatty acids. Supplements play a vital role in supporting the health of all cells and tissues in the body. It is impossible to get all our nutrients from foods because of how terribly adulterated our food sources have become.

Our processed foods have had the vitamins stripped away from them; fortifying these foods does not add the same amounts of vitamins back in that were originally taken out. Although convenient, these processed foods disrupt our bodily functions, all for the sake of economics and prolonging shelf-life; not for the sake of human life.

As an example, a 1982 study reported that pasteurization denatures enzymes, decreasing the bioavailability of the folic acid and other nutrients found in raw milk. Let's look at refined simple carbohydrates as another example.

This "refining" process removes nutrients from foods, but it also concentrates the sugar within the simple carbohydrate food. This causes excessive stress on the pancreas, the organ responsible for removing sugar (glucose) from the bloodstream and moving it into muscle cells to be burned as fuel. Pancreatic stress manifests as insulin over-secretion, causing (for a while, anyway, until it gives up) low blood sugar swings with a vicious cycle of blood sugar over-shooting and under-shooting as the body tries to auto-regulate. Is it any wonder why the incidence of diabetes continues to grow in this country?

The "refining process" also removes most of the fiber necessary to slow the release of the sugar into the system; slow release of sugars eases the burden on the pancreas. Poor soil conditions, herbicides, pesticides, genetically-modified foods, (GMF), preservatives, flavorings, coloring agents, bleaching agents, emulsifiers, food additives, fake sugars and trans-fats have replaced the "real" foods to which past generations were accustomed.

Our bodies do not know how to metabolize these "fake" foods. In turn, over time, the consumption of these foods gradually leads to symptoms that manifest themselves as the chronic illnesses and diseases that are plaguing us in the 21st Century.

*S*upplementing our diets with the proper amounts of the right nutrients will enhance the function of the immune, reproductive, digestive and circulatory systems. It will also *decrease* the risks of other diseases and health ailments such as depression, headaches, chronic fatigue, memory loss and anxiety.

If you are still skeptical about the use of supplements, consider the effects of vitamin C deficiency in the following story.

James Lind, a Scottish physician in the 1700s, discovered that one of the greatest threats to sailors of earlier centuries was an increased weakness of their blood vessels, bleeding and death. Many sailors did not return from their trips, due to scurvy, a condition caused by vitamin C deficiency.

Through a simple experiment, Dr. Lind proved that providing sufficient quantities of lime and lemon juice to the sailors could prevent bleeding and blood loss. He saved millions of lives by feeding the sailors these fruits. Unfortunately, it took 40 more years to put the discoveries by Dr. Lind into practice and to distribute limes to the British sailors. To this day, British soldiers are called "Limeys" because these fruits restored their health.

Even today, there is controversy over the use of vitamin C and its role in optimal health. This vitamin is the cornerstone to good health in that it is responsible for the production of collagen and connective tissue, and for optimum stability of the blood vessel walls.

OTHER SUPPLEMENTS FOR HORMONE BALANCE

B complex (25-100 mg daily) supports the liver so it can break down estrogen. Stress has a tendency to drain your body of vitamins, and many women experience an inordinate amount of stress during the menopausal phases, so it is advisable to consume additional B vitamins. B6, (pyridoxine) in particular, plays an important role as an enzyme co-factor that transforms one hormone to another.

Folic Acid (B9), (400 to 800 mcg daily) which is the form of folate in supplements, is known to play a role in breaking down homocysteine. High levels of homocysteine, an amino acid that is a byproduct of metabolism in the blood, are found in people who experience depression. Mood swings and depression are included in the cascade of symptoms women suffer during the menopausal process. Fresh vegetables are a good source of folic acid, so it appears that increasing fresh vegetables could drastically reduce depression.

Vitamin C (at least 3,000 mg daily, taken throughout the day), is recommended for purposes mentioned earlier; 5,000-10,000 mg per day if you feel a cold coming on, have allergies, or are under undue stress.

Linus Pauling, Ph.D., the great scientific maverick who studied chemistry, physics and mathematics, is best known for receiving the Nobel Prize in Chemistry in 1954 and the Nobel Peace Prize in 1962. He is also known as the greatest pioneer of vitamin C research. According to Pauling's research, this vitamin's versatility in illness prevention arises from its role in the manufacture of collagen, the protein that gives shape to connective tissues and strength to skin and blood vessels. He recommends at the first sign of a cold symptom or infection, 4-10 grams/day until bowel tolerance (loose bowels) is reached. That amount is effective in fighting both bacterial and viral infections.

Vitamin E (400-1,600 IU in d-alpha tocopherol form daily) helps to decrease mood swings, menstrual pain, hot flashes and anxiety. We are finding out of late, that toco-trienols are much more powerful than tocopherols. A newly discovered toco-trienol called di-desmethyl-tocotrienol, or P25, is obtained through a special molecular distillation of rice bran oil. P25 toco-trienols are not only far superior to the d-alpha tocopherol, but they might even replace your cholesterol-lowering drugs as well. As a bonus, double-blind, placebo-controlled human studies have shown that the toco-trienol form of vitamin E lowers cholesterol, improves LDL:HDL levels, and provides general heart-protection. This is an alternative to statin drugs, without the side effects.

Quercetin (50-300 mg daily) is consumed to reduce excessive estrogen levels while helping to maintain good cholesterol levels and proper digestion. It is also a potent antioxidant that protects the cells from "free radical" damage. Free radicals are single molecules with an unpaired electron in their outer electron ring. They are constantly created in body metabolism by pollutants such as smog, chlorine, food additives, radiation, benzene, and cigarette smoke.

Essential fatty acids (EFA) from flaxseed. (2-4 Tbsp.) per day of ground flaxseed is preferable over flaxseed oil due to oil having a propensity to become rancid. Flaxseed reduces several symptoms, such as breast tenderness, bloating, menstrual cramps, and pain due to endometriosis. It has been known to be extremely effective for women who have suffered from breast cancer. EFAs protect joints and bones, are required for the normal development of the brain and its function, and are also necessary for the eyes, adrenal glands and reproduction. Flaxseed is best used on cereals, in yogurt or in nutritious shakes.

Bioflavonoids (500-2,000 mg daily) slow down the overall activity of estrogen and work very well with vitamin C to reduce histamines and inflammation. Flavonoids are natural chemicals found in plants, fruits and vegetables and belong to the antioxidant-rich polyphenol group. Research has shown that flavonoids have many health promoting properties. They have been known to improve loss of memory and poor concentration, which women struggle with during phases in their cycle. They keep the heart healthy by preventing blood clots. They protect against oxidation of LDL (bad) cholesterol and have been effective in lowering high blood pressure.

Probiotics are better known as friendly bacteria. They are the good bacteria found in the intestines and other parts of the body. Lactobacillus acidophilus, lactobacillus bulgaricus, and bifidobacterium bifidum are the most common. *Everyone* (yes, I mean everyone), should be taking some form of probiotics today in order to protect the body from bacteria found in our foods and water. Live bacteria or cultures are found in yogurt in the grocery store, but have a very short shelf life. And don't depend on getting much good bacteria from this source, as many of the fruited yogurts contain more sugar than beneficial bacteria. Consuming a plain flavored organic yogurt is a better choice, if you enjoy yogurt; however, the best way to consume a good probiotic is in a supplement form in which thousands to billions of organisms are condensed into capsule form. Look for supplements that are refrigerated in order to sustain the potency of the good bacteria.

Digestive Enzymes. Good hormone balance begins in the gut. Following the western diet starves our bodies of enzymes. Heartburn, stomach upset, gas, bloating, indigestion and constipation are common complaints from many women. Failure to regularly eliminate body wastes is one of the most frequent causes of illness; exercise, proper food and other good habits are better than drugs to cure constipation. Using Zantac,

Prevacid, Tagamet or Tums is not going to solve the problems. These drugs only treat the symptoms and mask the underlying causes. Yet women are so terribly frustrated and uncomfortable with the pain, they reach for the quickest and easiest solution, not realizing the harm they are doing.

These drugs decrease the amount of acid the stomach makes, yet stomach acid is the body's first line of defense against stomach bugs like parasites and H. pylori. What the stomach really needs is more acid!

Heartburn, for example, is not caused by the production of too much acid. Acid Reflux, which is sometimes referred to as Gastroesophageal Reflux Disease (GERD) or reflux esophagitis, (the medical term for heartburn) is an inflammation of the esophagus. This inflammation is caused by regurgitation of the stomach contents, thus named acid reflux. The condition is more commonly recognized by its symptom of heartburn which reportedly affects 10 percent of American adults every day. It occurs when food is not digested quickly enough and falls back into the esophagus. The stomach needs more acid in order to move food out.

Some good digestive enzymes are amylase, protease, lipase, cellulose, papaya and pineapple enzymes (papain and bromelain). These are best taken after meals.

Black Cohosh or *Cimicifuga racemosa* (80-160 mg daily of standardized extract), is known to decrease hot flashes, night sweats, headaches, mood swings, vaginal dryness, heart palpitations, sleep conditions, and depression. Since it does not have estrogenic action and does not contain phytoestrogens, it is safe for use in patients with a history of breast cancer.

Black Cohosh is the leading herbal therapy for hot flashes in Europe. With tall spikes of brilliant white flowers and a gnarled, resin-scented root, black cohosh — the name is believed to be Indian in origin — grows wild in the deciduous forests of the eastern United States. American Indians have used it as a folk remedy for centuries. Black cohosh is the most studied herbal supplement for menopausal symptoms.

RemiFemin, one of the more popular products used by women in the U.S., is a unique extract of black cohosh and has been the subject of more than 20 clinical trials, as well as open clinical monitoring trials in physicians' practices. All studies reviewed in the *Annals of Internal Medicine* report were conducted using RemiFemin. In addition to the studies reviewed, there have been two reports published in 2002 confirming that RemiFemin is safe, effective and estrogen-free.

The Cherokee relied on alcoholic spirits of black cohosh root to treat rheumatism, and grounded the root into teas to treat constipation and fatigue; the Algonquins used it for kidney trouble. By 1849, the newly formed American Medical Association was describing black cohosh as useful for "the debility of females attendant upon uterine disorder." Taking 40-80 mgs. of a standardized extract of black cohosh, twice daily, is recommended for relief of menopausal symptoms.

Calcium (600-1,200 mg daily). The majority of calcium is found in our bones and teeth. Since bones are constantly being made and unmade, there is a constant need for calcium. All women should be taking calcium at a 2:1 ratio of calcium to magnesium. Without the assistance of magnesium, taking more calcium is for naught. Calcium citrate is better overall than calcium carbonate, as it has a better absorption rate when stomach acid is low. High levels of calcium can be found in leafy green vegetables, broccoli, tofu and black-eyed peas.

Magnesium (600-1,200 mg daily). Magnesium assists in calcium absorption and improves energy production in the heart, coronary arteries, and lowers blood pressure. It also is known to decrease menstrual cramping and has been highly effective in terminating an acute migraine headache.

Nutritional Balance

Our culture struggles desperately with the idea of "balance". All too often it is the all or nothing theory, or if something is good in small amounts, then larger amounts must be better. A good example of this is the variety of fad diets that have been luring millions of Americans into a false sense of good health. Low carbohydrates, high protein, all fruit juicing, low fat, low sugar, acidity versus alkaline, to name a few, has Americans hopping from one fad to another and spending millions of dollars in hopes of losing weight.

Sorry to disappoint everyone. In the long run, these diets rarely work, because it's a lifestyle change, not only diet, that constitutes success. Furthermore, individuals have different needs, so there is no one-diet-fits-all program.

Oh, sure, when starting a new diet, weight loss is always quick and quite evident. The true test is time and this is where most of these diets fail. There is no silver bullet when it comes to good health, although some experts are trying their best to prove otherwise. To gently assist your body nutritionally as it moves through the menopausal cycles, there are many foods that can make a noticeable difference for the better. The importance of nutrition in health and disease is too often overlooked.

Acidity versus Alkalinity

There has been a lot of talk lately about the pros and cons of consuming acidic foods versus alkaline foods. Everyone's metabolic processes are different, so each person's body will respond differently to particular foods. The key is the correct balance of carbohydrates, proteins and fats, which in turn relates to the balance of an acidic and alkaline environment.

For those who are overly acidic, eating more carbohydrates will make you feel better. For those who produce more alkaline, a diet of more protein will make you feel better. Based upon this information alone, you can determine what foods will make you feel better.

Undeniably, the consumption of hearty, nutritious foods plays a major role in your health. Vegetables, whole grains, cold water fish (such as salmon, mackerel and tuna), poultry, nuts, legumes and good melons (such as pineapple and papayas), will help you strike the balance you are looking for. *"Let thy food be thy medicine"* is a well known tip Hippocrates gave us long, long ago. Your body will tell you what it needs.

BUY ORGANIC

Organic foods may be unaffordable for some, but what are you spending on healthcare insurance, over the counter and prescribed drugs, doctor visits and other risky approaches that are supposed to assure good health? You will either pay now or pay later.

For those who find these foods expensive, start out by buying just a few items at a time while adjusting other lifestyle behaviors. Join a co-op whereby groups of people work together to buy directly from the farmer. Many neighborhood communities are creating this trend. If you do not have a co-op in your neighborhood, perhaps it's time you started one.

Organic foods are grown without xeno-hormones (hormones not found in nature) pesticides, herbicides, fungicides and insecticides. These hormones wreak havoc with your body's ability to produce the necessary hormones that balance the endocrine glands. They are neither genetically modified nor devoid in nutrients like many of the non-organic foods.

Scientific studies have shown that organic farming produced significantly higher flavonoids (plant by-products known to protect plants from insects, bacterial and fungal infection and photo-oxidation) in fruits and vegetables than conventional farming. In fact, previous studies indicated that conventionally farmed foods had higher levels of nitrates and synthetic pesticides and fewer total solids than organic foods.

NATURAL PROGESTERONE

Progesterone is a hormone, made by the corpus luteum that is responsible for the survival of the fertilized egg and the fetus throughout gestation. This is how progesterone got its name, in that it promotes a healthy gestation period. It is also the hormone that increases at the time of ovulation, increasing the sense of libido, thus creating the urge to procreate. Mother Nature was masterful at creating such a beautiful plan for the time sperm meets egg.

To drive home the point of natural progesterone's miraculous properties, a study was conducted early last year using injections of a progesterone-type hormone, 17-alpha-hydroxprogesterone caproate or 17P, a derivative of the hormone progesterone to prevent premature births. It was reported that pre-term births in women with a history of giving birth early were reduced by 34 to 42 percent, as reported by Paul J. Meis, M.D., of Wake Forest University Baptist Medical Center. "The evidence of this treatment's effectiveness was so dramatic, the research was stopped early," said Meis, the national principal investigator and a professor of obstetrics and gynecology at Wake Forest. "This drug is readily available and can be used by doctors to improve outcomes for mothers and babies."

If women used natural progesterone crème during pregnancy, there would be no need for injections, as natural progesterone allows the embryo to survive and aids in the development of the fetus throughout the pregnancy.

Under normal birthing circumstances, during the third trimester, progesterone is produced at the rate of greater than 300 mg/day which is far more than any other hormone produced. This is why women appear to have a glow about them prior to delivery.

On the dark side, however, when natural progesterone is converted into a synthetic form, (i.e., Provera) its ingestion actually blocks the binding of the woman's naturally-produced progesterone. This inability to bind to the receptor sites results in a profound and real progesterone deficiency. In fact, the anti-progesterone compound, RU-486, better known as the morning-after pill, blocks the level of progesterone, which will result in the loss of the embryo (abortion).

The use of natural progesterone crème and its efficacy for assisting women through the menopausal cycle is likely to be one of the greatest scientific breakthroughs in women's health. Thanks to Dr. Lee, several books have been written about this miraculous hormone.

Through clinical observations and having sifted through mounds of research, Lee extracted scientific evidence substantiating the need and use of natural progesterone crème. Because the majority of women are estrogen dominant, the need for progesterone in its natural state begins to provide the hormonal balance necessary to lessen the symptoms women experience during menopause. Use of this crème has been shown to produce many other medicinal benefits, as well.

THE FACTS

Knowing the physiological changes that occur during the menopausal cycle will help women understand why the need for natural progesterone is so important. The first order of business is to clear up the misconceptions that have run rampant for the past 50 years.

Women continue to produce hormones, namely estrogen, even after menstruation ceases. The medical mentality has preached the need for estrogen replacement and other synthetic hormones because the cycle of menopause has been classified as a deficiency disease. Women continue to make estrogen, although they make less than when the lining of the uterus is preparing for pregnancy. A woman's body makes estrogen from androstenedione in her fat cells.

Levels of progesterone, on the other hand, fall precipitously to almost zero during menopause and, sometimes, even before menopause. Combine this action with poor diets consisting of processed foods, the lack of vitamins and falling hormone levels, and what you get is one unpredictable, mood swinging female! And some of these moods are not so nice. There are many other symptoms that occur during this time also, such as hot flashes, vaginal dryness and weight gain.

The logical approach is to bring the hormones back into balance through a multi-faceted approach led by the use of natural progesterone crème. The following guidelines will outline the use of natural progesterone crème throughout the phases of a woman's life.

Natural Progesterone Crème Guidelines

PMS Sufferers

To start, use a full two-ounce jar or tube beginning on day 12 to day 26 of your menstrual cycle. (Day 12 is determined by using the first day of menstruation as day one). Use a dab in the morning and a dab in the evening in a crescendo pattern (a little bit more each day) and use a much larger dab the last few days. Because PMS is exacerbated by many contributing factors, (such as stress, diet, and sleep deprivation), adjustments may be needed as lifestyle balance begins to occur. As the body begins to adjust and symptoms decrease, less crème will be needed.

MONTHLY MIGRAINE SUFFERERS

Begin using natural progesterone crème on day 16 to day 26, about 10 days before menstruation begins. When you start to feel the "aura" right before the migraines begin, apply a dab (1/4 to 1/2 teaspoon) to your temple area or neck, every three to four hours until symptoms decrease.

MENSTRUATING WOMEN

Apply a dab (1/4-1/2 teaspoon) of natural progesterone crème to your wrists, inner arms, neck area, and the bottom of your feet (if they are not callused), once in the morning and once in the evening beginning on day 12 through day 26. Day 12 is determined by using the first day of menstruation as day one.

FOR INFERTILITY

Apply a dab (1/4-1/2 teaspoon) of natural progesterone crème to the areas listed above in the morning and in the evening beginning on day five and ending on day 26. Day 5 is determined based upon the fifth day of menstruation. Using the progesterone crème prior to ovulation effectively suppresses ovulation. After a few months of this regime, STOP. If you still have follicles left, they seem to respond to a few months of suppression with fervor and the successful maturation and release of an egg.

PREMENOPAUSAL WOMEN (IRREGULAR CYCLES)

Apply a dab (1/4-1/2) of natural progesterone crème to the areas listed above in the morning and in the evening beginning on day 12 through day 26. Day 12 is determined by using the first day of menstruation as day one. If menstruation begins before day 26, stop using the crème and resume beginning on day 12 of the next cycle using the first day of menstruation as day one. (There could be a great deal of irregularity during this time; therefore, menstruation may begin to decline anywhere from 5-10 years prior to menopause).

MENOPAUSAL WOMEN (NON-MENSTRUATING)

Apply a tiny dab (1/8-1/4 teaspoon) of natural progesterone crème to the areas listed earlier for 24–26 days. It's easiest to begin on the first day of the month and end on day 24, 25 or 26. Take a 5-6 day break and begin on the first day of the next month again. Always try to use a dab in the morning and in the evening. This pattern is the closest to replicating your own body's production of progesterone.

WOMEN WHO HAVE HAD A HYSTERECTOMY (SURGICAL MENOPAUSE) - REMOVAL OF THE UTERUS AND OVARIES

Hysterectomy means that all ovarian hormones are lost. Apply a dab (1/4-1/2 teaspoon) to the areas listed above in the morning and in the evening for 24–26 days, then take a break for about 5 days and resume the 24-26-day cycle. Because all the hormones are lost, some women need assistance with a low dose estrogen (bio-identical hormone) along with testosterone. The best way to determine this need individually is to take a saliva hormone assay test. This will be discussed later in the chapter. Measuring the hormones through the blood is not as accurate. Work with a healthcare professional who understands physiology, in order to achieve hormone balance.

WOMEN WITH FIBROCYSTIC BREASTS

Apply a dab (1/4-1/2 teaspoon) to the areas listed above in the morning and in the evening while ovulating (usually day 12-14 using day 1 as the first day in the cycle) and ending on day 26 or a day or two before menstruation begins. This will usually result in normal breast tissue within three to four months.

WOMEN WITH OSTEOPOROSIS

Apply a dab (1/4-1/2 teaspoon) to the areas listed above in the morning and in the evening starting on day 12 using day one as the first day of the calendar month and ending on day 26 for women who are still menstruating. For women who are not menstruating, apply a dab (1/4-1/2 teaspoon) in the morning and in the evening beginning on day one and ending on day 25 or 26 and resume on day one again of the next month.

These recommendations are based upon a two-ounce jar/tube of crème that contains a total of 960 mg of progesterone. This equates to 40 mg per 1/2 teaspoon, 20 mg per 1/4 teaspoon and 10 mg per 1/8 teaspoon. (*These recommendations are reprinted with permission from What Your Doctor May Not Tell You About Breast Cancer, John R. Lee, MD, David Zava, Ph.D., and Virginia Hopkins, 2002*).

There are a variety of good natural progesterone crèmes on the market. To be certain you are using an effective dose, make sure the two-ounce jar/tube/pump contains a minimum of 960 mgs. of natural USP progesterone. Using a crème with the most natural ingredients is also recommended. Read the label to be sure you know what you are buying. See the back of the book under *Resources* for the names of some progesterone crèmes that contain the recommended doses.

Please remember, for the best results it is very important to consume a proper diet, exercise, and consume proper minerals and vitamins to complement the usage of natural progesterone crème. This approach is multi-faceted.

Incorporating these lifestyle changes gradually and over time creates a therapeutic and positive impact. This approach is not like a drug that may have an immediate effect. This may take a little while, as you are assisting your body back to a state of balance. Be patient and watch the results.

TESTING HORMONE LEVELS FOR ACCURACY

Before the sophistication of diagnostic tools and tests, we relied on symptoms to tell us how to treat conditions. The symptom approach is a very powerful tool and is still used with a great deal of accuracy. This approach is a good rule of thumb, particularly when combined with the availability of testing.

Measuring hormone levels has always been done through the blood. However, through experimentation and testing, we have discovered that saliva is a much more accurate means of measurement.

In one research study conducted by Choe, JK, et al, the percentage of progesterone found in the saliva was 40 to 50 percent protein-bound, whereas only 3 to 6 percent was found in the plasma. Another study was conducted to measure the levels of progesterone and cortisol in saliva in women with post-partum blues. Salivary progesterone levels peaked before delivery and fell by day ten postpartum. There was no correlation between postpartum blues and progesterone levels in plasma, thus showing the difference between saliva and plasma measurements.

Many physicians do not use saliva as a means to test hormones, most likely because they are not familiar with the literature and were never taught to do so. However, this is changing due to women who are informing them of better methods.

A certain percentage of steroid hormones escape the blood-stream and become free or "bioavailable". Saliva testing is the most reliable way to measure the free, bioavailable hormonal activity—hormones actually doing their job at the target tissues of the breast, uterus, brain, and skin. It is at the tissue level that hormones do their work, or if unbalanced, do their damage. There is a strong correlation between bioavailable levels of steroid hormones in saliva and the levels of steroid hormones measured in blood tests. Most standard blood tests do not measure bioavailable hormone levels.

A local practicing administrator who manages a large thriving OB/GYN practice in the Tampa Bay Area has informed me that this method of saliva testing has always been an approved method of testing. The Current Procedural Terminology (CPT) codes, which are the official guidelines for pathology and laboratory testing, state the following: *"Many lab tests can be performed by different methods. To choose the correct code, carefully review code descriptions as well as any notes"*. Only if physicians are informed, will they know to use *saliva* instead of the *blood* as a means of measuring hormone levels accurately. Some healthcare plans are beginning to take notice of this changing practice. Be sure to share this information with your doctor.

The challenge is to find a lab that knows how to do the test. Currently, there are not many labs set up to do this type of testing. It is easy enough, however, to send off a saliva sample in the kits that are made available from these labs. See the back of the book under *Resources* for the name and location of labs, that provide testing and consultation.

Informed healthcare practitioners who are working with women to manage the change of life cycles naturally are using saliva testing as a complement to their assessment of symptoms. They are finding it to be an invaluable tool. Saliva testing not only determines the level of hormones, but it is also able to identify other imbalances that may manifest into other conditions and illnesses. It can also validate that the amount of natural progesterone crème (or other bio-identical hormones) you are currently using is in the proper dosage.

If you are interested in testing all the steroid hormone levels (progesterone, cortisols, estrogens DHEA and testosterone), share this information with your personal physician. There is no reason to test the blood for hormone measurement unless the doctor is looking for other pathology.

It is strongly recommended and confirmed that a more natural approach to managing the changes a women experiences throughout her lifecycle is safer than using synthetic drugs to balance hormones. Rest assured, you are on your way down the healing path when you assist the body with a more natural and balanced approach.

Keep your healthcare practitioners informed by sharing this information with them. The labs listed under *Resources* in the back of the book are also available to answer your questions.

*"No matter who says what, you should accept it
with a smile and do your own work."*
—*Mother Teresa*

4

THE BREAST CANCER INDUSTRY...
THE DARK SIDE OF HALF TRUTHS

ON THE AMERICAN CANCER SOCIETY'S (ACS) web page under the title, Making Strides Against Breast Cancer, there is not one reference to *prevention*. It does state that the disease will strike more than 200,000 times this year and will claim more than 40,000 lives.

The goal of *Making Strides* is to raise money for awareness, foster camaraderie, raise funds for breast cancer research, patient services, education and advocacy. Yet, there are no references to *prevention*.

After navigating the site thoroughly, I found the following statement: *"We do not know how to prevent breast cancer but it is possible that a female of average risk for breast cancer might decrease her risks somewhat by changing those risk factors that can be changed, such as giving birth to several children and breast feeding them for several months, avoiding alcohol, exercising regularly and maintaining a slim body."*

How disappointing, since we do have strong evidence—evidence that I will discuss later—that tells us how to prevent breast cancer. Unfortunately, this institution (ACS) that has branded itself as being the foremost leader in breast cancer information is also perceived by most women as being the best place to obtain up-to-date information.

There are many services the ACS provides that are valuable and useful; however, when it comes to education and *prevention*, it is twenty years behind the research. What is most troubling is that as a research institution, their number one goal, other than to treat disease or attempt to cure it as they claim, should be to inform women about how to *prevent* the disease. Wouldn't you rather *prevent* a disease from occurring in the first place than treat it once it has been diagnosed? Evidently, not many think so.

The National Cancer Institute (NCI) claims it is committed to *prevention*, but its budget and policy priorities reflect anything but. Set by Congress, NCI's budget in 2004 was $4.74 billion. Although this amount is a mere 3.3 percent increase over the 2003 year's budget, there are more contributions made by private donors. The National Institutes of Health (NIH), which is overseen by NCI, will provide an additional $909 million for cancer research through the National Institute of Environmental Health Sciences and other agencies.

The Department of Veterans Affairs will most likely spend over $457 million in 2003 for research and *prevention* programs. The Center for Disease Control (CDC) will contribute about $314 million for outreach and education, and the Pentagon will contribute about $249 million for nearly 500 peer-reviewed grants to study breast cancer, prostate and ovarian cancer. This budget does not include other generous contributions from fund raisers, other charities and research hospitals that total close to $2 billion.

Finally, The Tufts Center for the Study of Drug Development estimates that drug companies will invest about $7.4 billion, or about one-quarter of their annual research and development budget for products to treat cancer and metabolic and endocrine diseases. This is almost twice as much as NCI's entire budget in 2004.

On top of all of this we have generated a total of 1.56 million papers over the past 30 years in scientific journals. We, as Americans, have spent through taxes, donations and research and development close to $200 billion in inflation-adjusted dollars since 1971 in hopes of finding a "cure" for cancer.

The incidence of breast cancer is rising in epidemic proportions today. Except for skin cancer, breast cancer is the most commonly diagnosed cancer among American women. It is second to lung cancer as the leading cause of cancer-related death. According to NCI, breast cancer incidence rates increased by more than 40 percent from 1973 to 1998. In 2000, approximately 182,800 women were diagnosed with breast cancer.

In 2003, an estimated 211,300 new cases of invasive breast cancer were diagnosed among women and 39,800 women will have died of this disease. If detected early, the five-year survival rate for localized breast cancer is 97 percent. A report released in June 2004 from the Institute of Medicine at the National Academies in Washington has stated the same statistic as the ACS, that more than 200,000 new cases of breast cancer will be diagnosed in 2004 and more than 40,000 women will die from it.

Although many statistics claim that the incidence and prevalence of breast cancer is decreasing, the reality of the situation is that the incidence of breast cancer is steadily rising, and the numbers are appalling. Overall, cancer mortality has not improved since Richard Nixon declared war on cancer in the 1970s.

Today, popular ideas about breast cancer and its management are becoming outdated as research exposes their lack of merit. Sad to say, however, instead of unsuccessful treatment outcomes encouraging changes of common medical procedures, many practitioners are staunchly holding on to old ideas. A *Wall Street Journal* observer commented that the so-called targeted therapies, the current jewel in conventional oncology's crown, have not lived up to their promise. *"For the majority of patients, targeted therapies have been a disappointment,"* says Leonard Saltz, MD, of Memorial Sloan-Kettering Cancer Center, New York. "The word 'breakthrough' just doesn't fit".

And what do we get for all of this? The rate of Americans dying from cancer is about the same as in 1950 and 1970! The incident rate of cancer (all new cases) is expected to be one in two in men and one in three in women by 2020. And this is called progress?

PROFITS AND AWARENESS OVER PREVENTION

The detection, diagnosis and treatment of breast cancer is highly profitable in America. So what incentive is there to change the way our institutions look at breast cancer? Since 1985, October has been designated as National Breast Cancer Awareness Month. For years, women have donned pink ribbons, run races and walk-a-thons for "the cure", and religiously scheduled their yearly mammograms. Yet, only four decades ago the breast cancer rate was 1 in 20; today, it is 1 in 8.

Samuel S. Epstein, M.D., Professor of Environmental and Occupational Medicine at the University of Illinois, School of Public Health, has a different statistical view. Over recent decades, the incidence of cancer has escalated to epidemic proportions, now striking nearly one in every two men, and over one in every three women in their lifetimes. Even more disturbing is the recent recognition that this very high incidence of cancer is going to increase further still and, by the year 2050, will be doubling the current high incidence rate. How could it be then, that the cancer establishment still insists that we have turned the tide against cancer?

The Journal of the National Cancer Institute (JNCI) has commented that "private-practice oncologists typically derive two-thirds of their income from selling chemotherapy." This makes them financially dependent on increasing the acceptance and sale of expensive chemotherapeutic agents. They thereby have become advocates of the pharmaceutical companies rather than independent advocates for their patients' economic and medical interests. This situation is not conducive to making impartial treatment decisions. It also undermines the public's confidence in any positive statements made by the medical profession concerning the merit of chemotherapeutic drugs.

THE DEFINITION OF "PREVENTION"

Prevention appears to be a dirty word, and when it is discussed, it gets very little attention. Only a very small percentage of the National Cancer Institute's budget, as discussed earlier, is set aside for *prevention*. Yet, it is the only way to avoid the ravages of a disease that has changed thousands of women's lives forever, even if they do survive. Somewhere along the line over the years, the definition of *prevention* has been spun into meaning early detection and diagnosis. There is nothing further from the truth.

Prevention means to keep something from happening; to avert, or to anticipate or encounter in advance. *Early detection* is discovering or finding something hidden or obscure and *diagnosis* is the act or process of identifying or determining the nature of a disease through examination. Just because a woman may be diagnosed early and treated, does not mean the breast cancer is any less deadly.

DETECTION AND MAMMOGRAMS

Dr. Susan Love, a breast surgeon, testified before the Senate in 1991 and stated, *"We have spent a lot of time, energy, and money touting early detection and preserving it as if it were the answer. Unfortunately, we have misrepresented the situation through wishful thinking or just an attempt at simplification. We have acted as if all tumors go through progression from one centimeter to two centimeter[s] and on and on as if all tumors have the potential to be detected at a small size and therefore could be cured. I wish that were true. What we are dealing with is a combination of a tumor and an immune system. Some tumors are very aggressive and will have spread before they are palpable. Thirty percent of [the women with] non-palpable tumors are found to have positive lymph nodes. Some tumors are very slow growing and will not spread even though they have reached a large size."* She later notes, *"I think that any breast cancer large enough to be detected has already spread...The danger of cancer depends on the balance between the cancer and the ability of your body's immune system to fight it."*

As a result of the misinterpretation of *prevention and early detection,* women have been lured into comfortably believing that mammograms, as an example, are *the* preventive tool for breast cancer and depend on them too much, rather than taking an overall lifestyle approach.

Mammograms are a diagnostic tool. Of course it doesn't help that the media continues to send thousands of messages on a regular basis through the direction of our institutions, that every woman over forty should have an annual mammography. If this were, indeed, the way to prevent breast cancer, why are we seeing the incidence of breast cancer increasing? The effects of constant television-watching, the media and direct-to-consumer advertising of prescription drugs has created a nation of people who have become less able to separate truth from lies. The following comments may explain some of the reasons.

Mammograms fail to detect one fifth of all cancers in women under fifty. Having a clean bill of health from a mammogram does not necessarily mean a woman is cancer free. False positive results (a test result that is read as positive but actually is negative), cause women to be re-exposed to additional X rays and create an environment of further stress, even possibly leading to unneeded surgery.

Dr. Epstein says, "*While there is a general consensus that mammography improves early cancer detection and survival in post-menopausal women, no such benefit is demonstrable for younger women.*" Still, the ACS recommends annual or bi-annual mammography for all women ages forty to fifty-five or earlier.

As far back as 1974, Dr. Malcolm C. Pike, Ph.D., from the University of Southern California School of Medicine, warned NCI that a number of specialists had concluded that "giving a woman under age 50 a mammogram on a routine basis is close to unethical." Dr. Charles B. Simone, a former researcher at NCI, concurs. Hundreds of studies in peer-reviewed journals demonstrate that mammograms are risky and are often misdiagnosed or are incorrectly interpreted. One in four cancers in this age group is missed with mammography. "*Mammograms increase the risk for developing breast cancer and raise the risk of spreading or metastasizing an existing growth,*" says Dr. Simone.

Evidently, because many breast cancer cases are detected by mammograms, the current recommendations have been set for all women under 50.

Mammograms can be a useful tool, particularly for women over 50; however, this is only true when a qualified technician uses a reliable mammography machine with a skilled radiologist interpreting the results. There have been many misinterpreted mammograms that have caused a great deal of anguish for many women.

As counterintuitive as this may sound, radiologists Samuel Hellman and Jay Harris state that "detection of cancer at an earlier stage does not necessarily imply an improved cure rate."

The emphasis on mammograms has deterred women from doing self-breast examination, from thinking factually and rationally, and from learning about other lifestyle behaviors that can decrease their risk of breast cancer.

A recent report stated, *"Mammography saves lives and we need to figure out a way to get it to more patients more uniformly."* At the same time, the number of false-positive readings nearly doubled. The report further states that mammograms are not a perfect diagnostic tool, but no other technology has proved better at detecting breast cancer early.

Mammograms do *not* prevent breast cancer. Although mammograms lead to the discovery of smaller, earlier stage tumors, it still does not improve breast cancer survival rates over examination alone

And to complicate this emotional topic even more, last year a clinical trial in Canada reported that manual breast exams by trained medical practitioners were at least as likely to save lives as mammograms. This news upset the entire cancer establishment and scientists today are still arguing about what is right.

The benefits of annual screening of women age forty to fifty are, at best, controversial. Women's breasts can be and often are quite dense during this phase in life, which makes it more difficult to interpret the results of mammograms. There is also an abundance of good research showing that an excess of the female hormone estrogen is directly linked to breast cancer and that avoiding excessive estrogen can help prevent breast cancer.

THE AMERICAN CANCER SOCIETY'S RECOMMENDATIONS FOR EARLY BREAST CANCER DETECTION ARE AS FOLLOWS:

Women age 40 and older should have a screening mammogram every year, and should continue to do so for as long as they are in good health. Women should be told about the benefits, limitations, and potential harms linked with regular screening. Mammograms can miss some cancers. However, despite its limitations, mammograms remain an effective and valuable tool for decreasing suffering and death from breast cancer.

Mammograms for older women (over age 65) should be based on the individual, her health, and other serious illnesses. Age alone should not be the reason to stop having regular mammograms. As long as a woman is in good health and would be a candidate for treatment, she should continue to be screened with mammography.

Although these recommendations are considered the "gold standard", there is convincing evidence to believe otherwise as stated earlier. Based upon this evidence, I do not believe that all women should be mandated to have routine mammograms. For women in a very high risk category, however, such as family history of breast cancer or other risk factors discussed in the following chapter, this diagnostic tool should be considered. I also believe a woman's best protection against breast cancer is modifying her personal lifestyle habits to reduce risks.

If you are not comfortable with the idea of missing an annual mammogram, there is another diagnostic tool to consider called thermography. Unlike a mammography machine that uses radiation and painful compressions of the breasts, thermography uses a high-resolution camera that can read the temperature of your body and convert it into an infrared heat image that can be seen on a computer. This image is unique for each woman.

Studies have shown that an abnormal infrared image is the single most important indicator of high risk for developing breast cancer.

Thermography is able to detect the possibility of breast cancer much earlier, because it can image the early stages of angiogenesis. Angiogenesis is the formation of a direct supply of blood to cancer cells, which is a necessary step before they can grow into tumors of size.

To learn more about this technique you can contact the International Academy of Clinical Thermography at 650.361.8908 or 650.568.9292 or visit www.iact-org.org. This is a good starting point to find locations where thermography is performed, and to find a list of the risks and benefits of this diagnostic tool.

*C*learly, there is a medical crisis in the way we deal with breast cancer, both in its effect upon health and in its cost. Women find it very difficult to *"unlearn"* what they have been taught their whole lives. The powerful marketing efforts of conventional wisdom make it hard to separate what is "hype" from the practical and valuable information on these pages and other resources that place women's best interests first. It is much more comfortable to follow the illusions created by the hype than it is to face up to the harsh realities of truth.

The point is, we are fully aware of detection, diagnosis and treatment after eighteen years of "awareness" that has led us essentially to a dead end. And since *prevention* is not a profitable venture for the establishments, it is essentially ignored. Is this best for women? I say, "No."

*W*hat we really need to do is look ahead and shift our thinking to one of *prevention* and focus on the literature that supports this concept. Critics may argue that there is no substantial evidence to prove breast cancer is a preventable disease, but a body of science and scientists tell us otherwise. We are not in a position to wait another 20 years for the establishment to approve scientific studies of their liking. We must act immediately and take a pro-active approach.

This is not to say, however, that there is not a need for treatment and early detection. We do need early detection and treatment, but—even more—we need a national movement to embrace *prevention* if we want to decrease the incidence of breast cancer in this country. It's that simple.

THE CULTURAL LINE

Our culture is masterful at espousing ideology via media and other news venues without full disclosure. After the same message infiltrates for 30 to 40 years, similar to the HRT history, the consumer begins to believe it whether it is true or not. Nowhere is this more self-evident than in the knowledge about breast cancer.

A few years ago, TIME Magazine used their front page to feature an article about breast cancer. Much of the article was not particularly "new" or "good" news, but it sounded titillating and exciting. To me it was just a repeated message of the same old thing: surgery, radiation and chemotherapy—better known as slash, burn and poison. What may have prompted the writing of this article could have been an article that was published in *The Lancet*, a British medical journal, a few months prior.

In October 2001, Danish investigators Peter Gotzsche, M.D., and Ole Olsen, M.Sc., analyzed the seven major studies that form the foundation of the cancer establishment's mantra that annual mammography screening saves lives. These researchers determined that there is no reliable evidence that these screenings reduce mortality.

This information knocked the medical and science communities off their pedestals. Shortly thereafter, the National Cancer Institute agreed that the studies substantiating the efficacy of mammograms were seriously flawed and said it would rewrite policy statements to reflect this fact.

Eight major studies on mammography were reevaluated and researchers concluded that there *is* "fair evidence" that getting regular mammograms every year or two *could* reduce the chances of dying from breast cancer by about twenty percent over 10 years. *Could* reduce the chances? Where is the consistency? What and who is a woman to believe?

Prior to these reports, there have been ongoing arguments within the medical community about breast cancer screening. While the arguing continues, more women are diagnosed and die of this horrible disease, despite the fact that these supposedly "new" techniques are life savers. Is this not more of a reason to support *prevention* efforts?

As I mentioned earlier, after a constant message infiltrates a culture for 30 to 40 years, similar to the HRT history, the consumer begins to believe it whether it is true or not. It is quite telling here. The *TIME's* article did not mention prevention, nor did it discuss the risk factors or alternatives to diagnostic testing measures. Is this not a part of breast cancer education and research?

There are volumes of research that support all the previous information discussed so far, yet this information is rarely, if ever, written in mainstream publications. There is almost a sense of hostility toward *"prevention"* coming from established cancer experts and the medical establishment. Whenever the term *prevention* is mentioned, there is always a reason why it is worthless or there is no scientific evidence to support it. This is about as absurd as saying there is no way to prevent heart disease or diabetes.

Medicine, like any other professional field, is constantly evolving. What is good today, may not be good tomorrow. Yet the advancement often moves slowly and too cautiously, and oftentimes at the expense of human life. If we were to place as much emphasis on *prevention* as our institutions do on detection and treatment, we would have entirely different outcomes.

This may sound like pretty scary stuff, but it takes an open mind that can pick up knowledge along the way to help us move outside our security and comfort zones. Being open to new information will enable you to see the bigger picture and the deeper truth. For those who are hungry for the truth about breast cancer, the rewards are enormous and proportional to the effort of learning.

BREAST CANCER RISKS AND EVIDENCE

Dr. Epstein is an unpopular critic of the cancer industry. He persistently publishes documents that substantiate the direct link between pesticide residues and cancer and estrogen and cancer. He is one of many who emphasizes this scientific evidence; yet, his information is viewed with disdain by the medical establishment.

The ACS states on their website under the heading "Unproven Risks": "Pesticides play a valuable role in sustaining our food supply. When properly controlled, the minimal risks they pose are greatly overshadowed by the health benefits of a diverse diet rich in foods from plant sources." I do not consider the latest statistics, one out of eight women diagnosed with breast cancer, as minimal risks.

In 1993, Mary Wolff, M.D., and colleagues at Mount Sinai School of Medicine in New York, found that a relatively modest increase in levels of DDE (a breakdown product of DDT) resulted in a fourfold risk to women of developing breast cancer. Their conclusion: "Environmental chemical contamination with organochlorine residues may be an important causal factor in breast cancer." This is contrary to what the ACS is promoting.

There continues to be growing scientific evidence that supports the link between breast cancer and toxic chemicals found in the water, air, food and soil. This is not a local issue, but a global issue. Certain organochlorine chemicals, such as DDT, DDE, HCB, and dieldrin act like estrogen in a woman's body where they accumulate for years. These organic carcinogens act synergistically to induce breast cell proliferation.

Common household products, herbicides, pesticides, cigarette smoke, air pollution, prescription hormones, HRT, and many cosmetics are frequent sources of carcinogenic chemicals. Understand, however, that these are not the only risk factors linked to breast cancer. This disease is multi-factorial in nature, meaning there are several confounding factors that effect it. But, these carcinogens play a major role as risk factors of breast cancer.

Organochlorine pesticides are xenoestrogens (estrogens from an outside source). When reviewing risk factors associated with breast cancer, you will see that most of them are directly or indirectly associated with an excess of the female hormone estrogen.

Let us not forget about the results from the Million Women study and the Women's Health Initiative study that revealed the risks of using HRT. These studies show evidence of the estrogen connection. The more estrogen a woman is exposed to in her lifetime, the higher her risk for breast cancer. It is well established that estrogen is implicated in the formation of three cancers: uterine, germ cell and breast.

Use of HRT is associated with an increased risk of developing less common types of invasive breast cancer. The risk is also associated with duration of HRT use; the research team reported that postmenopausal women who used HRT for 5 years or less had an 80 percent higher risk of breast cancer than those who had not taken HRT. This risk rose to a 165 percent higher risk in those who had taken HRT for more than 5 years. The research was done at Northwestern University in Chicago and the Mayo Clinic.

Why did we have to wait until 2003 to stop a major study? Why are women still being prescribed HRT? Women need to stop and ask themselves why unpopular and contrary information that comes from resources other than popular medical institutions continues to be vehemently criticized. These scientists and institutions are equally qualified, if not more so, in reporting their scientific evidence. I believe the first step to scientific discourse is civility, not criticism coming from blind ignorance.

OLD HABITS DIE HARD…A LESSON IN HISTORY

Could it be that unless NCI or other medical institutions funded by NCI conduct research themselves, they are unwilling to accept research from other scientists that may not fit their mold? Often times, these *"wayward"* scientists are not given a public forum to discuss their results; while the larger institutions are granted such a forum. Is there a double standard here? Since when does one institution have a monopoly on medical research and information? If our scientists can't measure something, quantify it, or put it under a microscope, it does not exist to them. Some of the following examples could explain the disdain for change and why medical information is so often outdated before it gets into the hands of the consumer.

From the mid-19th century until the last 20 to 30 years, a high fiber/low animal fat diet was recommended by people who conventional institutions classified as charlatans and quacks. The concept of breast feeding by the LaLeche League, current studies of the efficacy of acupuncture, and discoveries in botanical medicine have been influenced and originated outside the walls of conventional medicine. Often, what is considered new is really quite old. We are coming full circle to understand that "old habits" are more valuable than we think.

Having said this, women have good reason to seek new routes and research beyond what is considered the "standard" body of information coming from established medical institutions. These institutions are not the only proper authority on health. With statistics as alarming as breast cancer, it is no wonder that more women are demanding full disclosure of information.

The conventional wisdom is that breast cancer is a normal part of life and treatments are available that save women's lives.

We must change this complacent thinking to confront and attack this epidemic of breast cancer. And please remember, being diagnosed with breast cancer is not usually a medical emergency. What I mean by this is that most women have a sufficient amount of time after a diagnosis to research treatment and other valuable health information before having to make any final decisions.

Jeanne Achterberg, PhD, senior editor of *Alternative Therapies Journal* said it beautifully: *"Change leaps forward episodically. It does not follow linear time, but rather bursts forth.*

Today, we are walking a razor's edge between skepticism and innovation." This skepticism is what is keeping the truth from women.

Conventional medicine narrowly focuses on diagnosis when it comes to treating chronic diseases and cancer and relies on drugs to kill the invader(s). Conventional medicine tries to kill the disease, hopefully, before it kills the patient.   In its fervor to find a magic bullet, which does not exist, the entire medical community has forgotten about *prevention* and healing. Our medical model has been reduced to a "one size fits all" and is the exact opposite of how individual women wish to be treated.

*R*obert W. Mahley, M.D., Ph.D., Professor, Pathology and Medicine, University of California San Francisco says it succinctly: *"There is no place for narrow-mindedness or protecting one's own turf if we are to solve complex diseases and advance prevention and treatment of disorders plaguing humankind."*

To augment Dr. Mahley's comments, Arthur Ponsonby, a British politician in 1928, stated profoundly, *"When war is declared, truth is often the first casualty."* Welcome to the war on cancer, ladies.

"You will observe with concern how long a useful truth may be known and exist, before it is generally received and practiced on."
—*Benjamin Franklin*

5

BREAST CANCER PREVENTION

THE WORLD HEALTH ORGANIZATION (WHO) issued a major report in 2003 that predicts cancer rates could increase by 50 percent by the year 2020. The report concludes that one-third of these cancers could be prevented by timely action with regard to smoking, diet and infection. The World Cancer Report is one of the most comprehensive global examinations of the disease to date. It provides clear evidence that *"healthy lifestyles and public health action by governments and health practitioners could stem this trend and prevent as many as one-third of cancers worldwide."*

The evidence of the importance of prevention continues to grow as we struggle to decrease the incidence of disease, which is an even stronger reason why women need to have this information in their hands to make good informed decisions.

Not all women have the same risk of developing breast cancer. While any woman can develop the disease, certain factors put some women at statistically greater risk. The following information will give you a snapshot of risk factors that can increase a woman's chance of getting breast cancer.

BREAST CANCER RISK FACTORS

HORMONAL FACTORS

- oral contraceptives, with early and prolonged use
- oral contraceptives during adolescence
- Hormone Replacement Therapy
- unopposed estrogen (without progesterone)
- removal of ovaries
- exposure to xenohormones and toxic chemicals

LIFESTYLE FACTORS

- obesity
- abortion
- excessive alcohol use
- tobacco use
- sedentary lifestyle
- dark hair dyes, with early or prolonged use

GENETIC FACTORS

- early puberty
- previous history of breast cancer.
- family history of breast cancer, particularly pertinent if the woman's mother or sister(s) had or have the disease
- late menopause
- age
- race

ENVIRONMENTAL FACTORS

- geography (living near an area polluted with industrial waste)
- exposure to radiation
- electromagnetic fields (EMFs)
- exposure to household chemicals
- workplace exposure to a wide range of carcinogens

DIETARY FACTORS
- insulin resistance
- diet high in animal fat
- low melatonin levels

DRUG FACTORS
- non-hormonal prescription drugs such as some antihypertensive drugs
- chemotherapy
- radiation (diagnostic and therapeutic)
- premenopausal mammography, with early and repeated exposure

WHAT CAN WOMEN DO?

There is hope. First of all, it's imperative that you not rely on only your personal physician for *all* the facts and information about breast cancer—it's your health issue and body! You do not need permission to research additional resources. Stretch outside the scope of conventional thinking. And if affirmation is what you need, the chapters in this book will provide it.

There is plenty of research available that provides full disclosure of information on breast cancer and prevention. This makes it nearly impossible for any one doctor to have all the answers. Find a medical authority who will talk to you and explore several options for prevention, treatment and healing. Find healthcare practitioners you can trust, i.e., those who have been successful in their practices and whose patients have had positive outcomes in regards to their treatment of health conditions. Make it your top priority to learn about *prevention*. Women *must not* be intimidated or pressured into doing something they do not really want to do.

A good doctor is much more than a well-trained technician or a scientist with a head full of facts. The practice of medicine remains, even in this scientific age, more art than science, more about human beings than technology. Indeed there is much to suggest that science and technology have somehow de-based the art of medicine and dehumanized the physician. The decision to apply or misapply that technology is often a judgment of the heart rather than the head. Caring and curing cannot be separated. If you're looking for a good scientific physician, one you can trust who will work with you, start by looking for a human being who cares about you.

There is no question that you can significantly reduce your risk of disease by getting regular exercise, eating a wholesome diet, maintaining a healthy weight, managing stress effectively, balancing your hormones naturally, avoiding the use of HRT and birth control pills, and avoiding artificial non-foods that are riddled with additives and preservatives.

Creating a healthy environment for your body will significantly reduce your risk of developing any degenerative illness or disease. These recommendations are good for everyone and they are based on pure simple logic. The information most women are lacking is what to do to *prevent* this devastating disease. Well, ladies and perhaps gentlemen, please continue reading to find the answers.

Breast Cancer Surgery and Survival Rates

Breast cancer surgery was performed at two major hospitals in London in 1976. During each surgery, a sample of blood was taken and saved to measure progesterone levels at the time of surgery. Higher levels of progesterone in these women correlated with longer survival rates. The survival record was reviewed 18 years after breast cancer surgery in node positive patients, i.e., in women whose cancer had already spread (was already metastasizing). In women with good progesterone levels at the time of their surgery, it was revealed that approximately 65 percent were still alive 18 years later, whereas only 35 percent of the women with low progesterone levels at the time of surgery were still alive.

Dr. Lee, a world renowned authority on women's health issues, has reported for many years that progesterone prevents breast cancer. If you already have breast cancer, progesterone can protect you against recurrence or late metastases.

Over the years, Lee treated many women who had mastectomies with progesterone. In the more than 20 years since he started recommending the use of progesterone, not one of the hundreds of women he treated has died of breast cancer. Think about these odds and compare them to normal post-mastectomy data. As Lee states, *"The goal of progesterone supplementation is to restore normal physiologic levels of bioavailable progesterone."* This is how Nature intended it to be.

NATURAL PROGESTERONE HAILS AGAIN

In a previous chapter, I discussed the miraculous value of the hormone progesterone; other studies are showing the value and protection factor of progesterone, too.

Results from a study conducted in 1981, reported that the incidence of breast cancer was 5.4 times greater in women with low progesterone levels than in women who had good progesterone levels. A Mayo Clinic study showed that women with a history of progesterone deficiency, as evidenced by symptoms such as irregular periods, had 3.6 times the risk of post-menopausal cancer.

Dr. K. J. Chang and his team of researchers conducted a study dividing women into four groups. Prior to biopsy, one group of women was given progesterone cream, one a combined estrogen, progesterone cream, one group estrogen and one a placebo. It was found that the levels of estrogen in breast cells had increased by 100 percent in those given estrogen cream. Progesterone levels in the breast cells had increased by 100 percent in those given progesterone cream. The levels of estrogen and progesterone had increased by 50 percent in those given the combination cream. There was no change in those given the placebo. In the biopsies, cell proliferation, which is the beginning of cancer, had increased by 230 percent in those given estrogen and reduced by 400 percent in those given progesterone. This clearly shows that progesterone reduces proliferation of cancerous breast cells.

The use of natural progesterone is well documented in the cases of breast cancer. Please tell every woman you know to explore this option if she has been diagnosed with breast cancer. Please be sure to visit the websites listed under *Resources* in the back of this book for more detailed information on this topic.

BREAST FEEDING

There is a 7 percent reduction of risk for breast cancer in women who were breastfed as babies. Breast feeding immunizes the mother as well as the infant. The *Lancet* reported these results and the analysis of 47 epidemiological studies considered to have covered over 80 percent of all the epidemiological data on breast cancer. The conclusion determined that a woman's risk of breast cancer decreases by 7 percent for every birth, three percent more for each year under twenty-eight years of age that she has another child, another 4.3 percent for every twelve months of her life that she breast-feeds, and another 23 percent if she was breast fed.

This information is often overlooked. Sadly, the idea of breast-feeding lost its allure long ago due to several reasons. By the end of the 1970s, 95 percent of babies were bottle-fed instead of breast-fed. Today, two-thirds of new mothers are now employed full-time, and only about 20 percent of all new moms in the U.S. breast-feed for six months or less.

According to Le Leche League International breast feeding statistics, about 70 percent of women begin to breast feed initially, and then this percentage drops down to 33 percent at around four to five months.

Baby formula has been marketed and promoted since the 1940s, marketing that has led many women to change their minds about breast-feeding. What is so fascinating about this social change is that between the years of 1940 to 1975, studies showed the greatest increase in the incidence of breast cancer. Convenience as a substitute for established healthful practices rarely outweighs original benefits.

A breast-fed baby's digestive tract contains *Lactobacillus bifidus*, a beneficial bacteria that prevents the growth of harmful organisms. Breast milk is always sterile and never contaminated by dirty bottles, which can lead to diarrhea in infants. Human milk also contains at least 100 more ingredients not found in formula. Babies are *not* allergic to their mother's milk, so there is no worry about allergic reactions.

As mentioned earlier, breast-feeding immunizes the mother as well as the infant. During breast-feeding, the mother is producing antibodies in her body that are transferring the collective memory of her immune system to her baby. And if you were breast-fed, the same thing occurred between you and your mother.

There are a few more benefits that should interest women regarding breast-feeding. Not only does it stimulate the uterus to contract back to its original size, sucking at the breast promotes good jaw development for the baby that encourages the growth of straight, healthy teeth. While breast feeding, the mother's levels of the hormone prolactin rise. This action of prolactin and estriol (a human estrogen released during pregnancy), cause the full maturation of breast milk duct epithelial cells, making the breasts less susceptible to future risk of breast cancer.

All the benefits mentioned above should be sufficient incentives to breast feed your baby. Health experts believe that increased breast-feeding rates would not only save lives, but would also save money on both infant formula costs and health-care expenditures.

Some researchers say that it is unrealistic to think Western women will revert to a lifestyle from two centuries ago. I strongly disagree. With all the benefits breast-feeding provides, it is this type of mentality that needs to be squelched. The idea has nothing to do with "going back in time." Understanding these benefits makes it clear why breast-feeding should be promoted as part and parcel of the entire birthing experience.

As more women begin to learn about the long term benefits breast-feeding provides, they will find a way to make it a priority. Women deserve to be aware of these choices. It is my hope that now that you are informed of the value of breast-feeding, you will decide to breast-feed, if and when the time comes.

For the Mom Who Works Outside the Home

Every mom is industrious, and when it comes to managing a family and home, she will always find a way to make things happen. With some advanced planning, breast-feeding can be incorporated into the working mom's schedule.

- Many women are able to take longer maternity leave

today, so it is a viable option to breast feed your baby for at least the first three to four weeks. It is not unusual for women to take six-month leaves that are even better for mom and the baby.

- A new mom can purchase or rent a good quality breast pump. Get started using it prior to returning to work so you are comfortable with the process.
- After pumping, store the milk in glass containers, not plastic. It's best to use the milk within 24 hours of pumping.
- Milk can be frozen but should be used within three months. Milk should be thawed in the refrigerator or under warm water.
- *Do not* boil the milk, nor use a microwave.
- Milk left over from a feeding should be discarded.
- Breast feed before leaving for work and as soon as you can when you return home.
- Lunch-time feedings are ideal, although often not possible.

Try to adjust your work schedule around your baby. It will be the best decision you ever made. For more information about breast feeding, contact the La Leche League International to find a convenient chapter near your home at (800/LA-LECHE) or 847.519.7730. Interested women and couples are invited to attend meetings at no charge.

CONTAMINANTS IN BREAST MILK

Recently, there have been reports about a particular type of flame retardant that has been discovered in human milk. Unfortunately, all babies born today have been exposed to ubiquitous toxins, as we do not live in a perfect world.

Several mothers in a study conducted by the Environmental

Working Group (EWG) were found to have high levels of polybrominated diphenyl ethers (PBDEs) in their breast milk. PBDEs are commonly used in upholstery, plastics, electronics, textiles, and construction materials. Lauren Sucher, spokeswoman for (EWG), stated, *"There was no trend, so it tells us it's a universal problem, that we can't blame behaviors for the exposure."*

Even though a small group of 20 women participated in this study, finding PBDEs in their breast milk, though not surprising, are profound. This certainly should not deter women from breast-feeding their babies. Breast milk is still the ideal means of providing the best nutrients and best start in life.

The results of this study confirm the need for prompt action to reduce children's exposure to toxic fire retardants in America. The EWG has made strong recommendations to the Environmental Protection Agency (EPA) to reduce pollutants in the environment.

The World Health Organization, the American Academy of Pediatrics, and other major health associations overwhelmingly support the importance of breast-feeding, even in a contaminated world. Greater marketing efforts should come from these organizations to emphasize the value of breast feeding.

Below are some helpful tips to avoid further exposure to toxins before, during and after pregnancy.

- Avoid smoking cigarettes and drinking alcohol since levels of contaminants have been found to be higher in those who smoke and drink alcoholic beverages.
- Be aware in purchasing homes and buildings that have been treated with pesticides for termites and/or older homes that might have lead-based paints.
- In general, eat a variety of foods low in animal fats; remove skin and excess fat from meats and poultry. Avoiding high-fat dairy products may reduce the

potential burden of fat-soluble contaminants.

- Increase consumption of grains, fruits and vegetables. Thoroughly wash and peel fruits and vegetables to help eliminate the hazard of pesticide residues on the skin. When available, eat food grown without fertilizer or pesticide application.
- Avoid fish such as swordfish and shark or freshwater fish from waters reported as contaminated by local health agencies.
- Limit exposure to chemicals such as solvents found in paints, non-water based glues, furniture strippers, nail polish, and gasoline fumes.
- Remove the plastic cover of dry cleaned clothing, and air out the garments in a room with open windows for 12-24 hours.
- Try to avoid contact with incinerator discharge, preserved wood, or produce grown near incinerators.
- For those in the workforce, attempt to avoid occupational exposure to chemical contaminants and seek improved workplace chemical safety standards for all employees, especially pregnant and lactating women.
- Encourage other family members to be sensitive to contaminant residue they may inadvertently bring into the home.

DIETARY CHOICES . . . GOOD FOR ALL

The recommendations in this section are not only important in the *prevention* of breast cancer, but overall, offer good advice to improve and sustain good health. Although there are hundreds of diets in the marketplace today that are screaming for your attention, here is some good, old-fashioned common sense that will not make you crazy and will make all the difference in the world in reducing your risk of disease.

Eat simple. Since diet may be responsible for more than 1/3 of all cancers, and because standard medical treatment of chemotherapy and radiation depletes valuable antioxidant enzymes and nutrients, nutritional support is imperative for healing and protection against further damage of healthy cells.

"He who eats till he is sick, must fast till he is well."
Hebrew Proverb

Food is fuel for the body. If you don't need much fuel, don't take it in. We overeat in this country and our gluttony has resulted in an epidemic of obesity. Over the years, consumers have minimized and ignored the dangerous health consequences of this behavior. Unspent fuel is either stored as fat or remains in the intestines where it will spoil and manifest itself in health problems.

In 2002, Americans spent approximately $115 billion on fast food, which exceeds the dollars spent on personal computers, new cars or higher education. Americans spent more than half their food budget on food and drinks consumed outside the home. For example, Coca-Cola Company statistics show that teenagers consumed 65 gallons of their soda pop, on average, in a year. On the other hand, overall consumption of vegetables has increased, but the increase has been in consumption of potatoes in the form of French fries. Eat more green, leafy vegetables, please. When you become aware of how our diet has changed, you will begin to see the direct link between lifestyle choices and the increased risk of illness and disease.

WHOLE FOODS

Whole foods are those that are organic, unprocessed and fresh in nature. They contain the greatest amounts of fiber, which assists in the digestive process and hormone balance. Whole foods include brown rice, whole wheat, millet, bulgur, legumes and foods in the carotene family, such as green leafy vegetables and yellow-orange fruits. Vegetables and fruits such as carrots, apricots, mangoes, yams and squash are a part of this family as well.

Various scientists have agreed upon an anti-cancer diet that includes peas, beans and lentils. This group of foods is collectively known as pulses or legumes. The World Cancer Relief Fund/American Institute for Cancer Research (WCRF/AICR) recommends legume consumption. The reasoning is that these foods are a good source of fiber, vitamins, minerals and other plant compounds that offer cancer fighting properties.

Forty-five to 60 percent of dietary calories should come from starchy or protein-rich foods of plant origin. The WHO recommends a daily consumption of 30 grams (about one ounce) of legumes, including nuts and seeds, to reduce the risk of heart disease and some types of cancer. Other studies have found that people who eat lots of beans enjoy a measure of protection against breast, prostate and colon cancer.

As a side note, countries with low rates of breast, colon, rectal and prostate cancer are those in which beans are a prominent staple of the diet. Countries with high rates of cancer tend to be those where bean/legume consumption is markedly lower.

The Bean Research Unit of the U.S. Department of Agriculture (USDA) loves to promote beans. When scientists studied twelve different types of beans, they found that these legumes contained many of the same antioxidants that are found in berries, fruits and wines that often cost more. What was also very interesting is that red and black varieties contained the highest amount of antioxidants compared to great northern white or cannellini beans. Eat your beans and enjoy. And don't be too concerned about a little flatulence, as the benefits outweigh the risks of social embarrassment.

THE VALUE OF FLAXSEED

Flaxseed is almost a perfect food, similar to the egg. Flaxseed's cancer-fighting power comes from its lignans, which, in your stomach, convert to estrogen-blocking agents. Flaxseed is especially rich in omega-3 fatty acids. It provides alpha linolenic acid (ALA), a substance the body converts to the heart-protective omega-3 fatty acids, also found in salmon, sardines, and mackerel. Saying this, however, does not mean you should overdo the consumption of flaxseed. America has adopted the mentality that if something is good, more of it is better. Don't buy this myth.

Flaxseed is the single most highly concentrated plant source of omega-3 fatty acids. When the body begins to absorb this ALA, a number of changes can occur on the surface. Skin becomes softer, hair becomes shinier and nails become stronger. But the real benefits occur inside the body.

Another great benefit of this seed is that it is extremely affordable. It costs literally pennies per ounce. In my opinion, no one should go without this miraculous seed. Flaxseed is a cancer fighter and it contains approximately one-third soluble fiber, which helps regulate blood glucose and lower cholesterol levels and two-thirds insoluble fiber, which can clean out the intestines. It also contains magnesium, iron, copper and zinc. One tablespoon of ground flaxseed contains only 36 calories.

At the University of Toronto, nutrition scientists, Dr. Lillian Thompson and Dr. Paul Goss, from Princess Margaret Hospital in Toronto, reported that flaxseed muffins had performed as well as the anticancer drug Tamoxifen in shrinking estrogen receptor-positive breast cancer tumors. These tumors account for two-thirds of all breast cancers.

This type of outcome and research is showing incredible promise, because the drug Tamoxifen is not as effective and safe as had been recently reported. Its side effects can be worse than the disease itself. In May 2002, the FDA suggested that the manufacturers of Tamoxifen include a warning label for fatal strokes, pulmonary embolisms and uterine malignancies.

At Duke University, in a pilot study published in the July 2001 issue of *Urology*, researchers slowed the growth of prostate cancer tumors with a dietary intervention of raw ground flaxseed. In this study, the men consumed 30 grams (3 tablespoons) of raw, ground flaxseed daily. The longer they stayed on the flaxseed enriched-diet, the better the results.

Although there is an ongoing debate within the scientific community regarding flaxseed and prostate cancer, studies have found flaxseed to be beneficial in the treatment and prevention of this form of cancer. Other studies have shown that flaxseed may actually increase the size of prostate tumors. Scientific differences of opinion exist everywhere, so it is wise to carefully research the topic before any serious decisions are made for treatment.

Before it is ground, flaxseed will remain fresh for eight months or more in a tightly covered container that is stored in a cool, dry place. Once it is ground, flaxseed should be refrigerated and used within a short period of time. Remember, these are oils, and they can go bad or rancid if not kept refrigerated. Less than 5 percent of the lignans make it to the oil during processing. Ninety-five percent remain in the ground seeds. Ground flaxseeds, therefore, are the most beneficial form to consume.

Gradually introduce flaxseed into your diet because it contains so much soluble fiber. Start with about 1 or 2 teaspoons a day and gradually increase the daily amount to 1 to 2 tablespoons per day as the body adjusts. Some experts suggest using up to 4 to 6 tablespoons per day, depending on personal needs and health conditions. Be sure to consume more fluids to help digest the extra fiber. Flaxseed can be easily incorporated into the diet by adding it to cereal, yogurt or a smoothie drink.

If you are not consuming flaxseed today, I strongly suggest that you begin. A benefit to using ground flaxseeds rather than the oil is two-fold. One, it is more economical, and two, the mucous portion of the flaxseed buffers excess acid, which makes it ideal for inflammation in the stomach and throughout the gastrointestinal tract. Eating flaxseed will help to promote normal cholesterol levels, improve your digestion, and help you feel better overall. It is considered the perfect food to consume for preventative measures.

REFINED CARBOHYDRATES

Americans love to consume breads, bagels, muffins, soda pop, other sweet drinks, candy, and chips. Unfortunately, these foods contain many calories and offer relatively no nutritional value. They keep blood sugar and insulin levels high and cause them to drop precipitously when withdrawn. This pattern can oftentimes turn into adult onset diabetes. Excess sugars and starches can also be converted into fats if exercise does not burn them as fuel; thus the body has an excess supply of glucose. This is not to say that you should not eat them; however, they should be consumed in moderation in order to provide a healthy balance overall.

FATS FOR ALL

We Americans have been misled to believe that *"all"* fats are bad, but there is nothing further from the truth. We need fat in our diets—the right kind of fats.

Dr. Raymond Peat, a biologist specializing in physiology and considered an expert in nutritional research, has worked with and studied progesterone and other related hormones since 1968. He believes that the sudden surge of polyunsaturated oils into the food chain after World War II has caused many changes in hormones. Peat has concluded that since the unsaturated oils block protein digestion in the stomach, we can be malnourished even while "eating well."

There are many changes in hormones caused by unsaturated fats. Their best understood effect is interference with the function of the thyroid gland. Unsaturated oils block thyroid hormone secretion, its movement in the circulatory system, and the response of tissues to the hormone. Coconut oil, on the other hand, is unique in its ability to prevent weight-gain.

Historically, polyunsaturated oils such as soybean oil have been used for livestock feed because they cause the animals to gain weight. The benefit is to the rancher at market, not to you the consumer. These oils are made up of what is known as long chain fatty acids—the kind of fatty acids that promote weight gain. Could this be a contributing factor to the current obesity epidemic in the U.S.? I think so.

Saturated fats found in beef and other feedlot animals should be consumed minimally. These animals have been dosed with pesticides and grains that have also been dosed with estrogens and other contaminated chemicals, unlike the grass fed to steers years ago. Excessively fatty diets encourage breast cancer by encouraging obesity. A higher incidence of breast cancer has been reported in obese women. Since body fat produces estrogen, there is a direct link.

The diet of previous generations included a good balance of essential fatty acids (EFAs), especially omega-3 fatty acids like those in flaxseed oil and deep-sea fish, and omega-6 fatty acids like those in safflower, sunflower, corn, canola, pumpkin and primrose oil, and sesame seeds and nuts. Omega-9 fatty acids are the monounsaturated fats, like those in olives and olive oils, avocados, walnuts, pecans, peanuts, almonds, filberts, macadamias, and cashews, all of which are very healthy for you. These fatty acids are called "essential" because our bodies cannot make them; therefore, we must get them from our foods.

Without fat, our bodies couldn't function. Fats are required for production of hormones to assist in the absorption of fat soluble vitamins like A, D, E and K and to help with oxygen transport and calcium absorption. Both the omega-3 and -6 fats play an important role in the body's production of prostaglandins, which are a special type of hormone produced throughout the body. They control most of your life-sustaining systems like heart function and the immune system.

Confusion exists because practically every fried food and snack food available has been cooked in soybean, corn, sunflower, safflower or canola oil that has been hydrogenated, a process that can eventually produce nerve tissue and cardiovascular damage. Hydrogenated oil (sometimes referred to as partially-hydrogenated) is a liquid vegetable oil that is bombarded with hydrogen molecules to make it more solid and thus protect it from oxidation and rancidity. These unnatural oils are used in all snack foods, such as margarines, chips, baked goods and frozen desserts. They wreak havoc with the body's hormones, thus creating a hormone imbalance by blocking the action of "good" EFAs.

Unfortunately, the consumer ends up with fats and oils that are the nutritional equivalent of other refined products —

demineralized, devitaminized, fiberless, empty calories that cannot be properly digested or metabolized and which rob the body of essential nutrients in the process.

In general, the refined oils mentioned above, are put through intensive processing that requires toxic chemicals during extraction from their vegetable, nut, or seed of origin. This process also leaves behind toxic residues. Sometimes, synthetic preservatives are added back in to replace the natural antioxidants destroyed in the processing. It's cheap to do and makes food tasty.

What is most important is a balance of these EFAs. With all the refined foods assaulted by this chemical process, particularly omega-6 EFAs, it is very difficult to achieve a balance. It has only been in the past year that eggs, an omega-3 rich food, have regained their prominence in the food chain. Many of the most popular seafoods, such as salmon, trout, catfish, shrimp and others, are now being farm-raised, dramatically lowering their omega-3 EFA content. Instead of a rich diet of algae, insects, or minnows, these farmed-raised fish eat omega-6 grains and grain by-products. This is just one more barrage of too many omega-6 EFAs.

Another overlooked factor that effects the imbalance of EFAs is over-the-counter and pharmaceutical agents. Although used with a great deal of confidence and with little thought of side effects, these agents disrupt the enzyme process that converts EFAs into prostaglandins. Consequently, there is an overabundance of omega-6 EFAs compared to the omega-3 and 9 EFAs.

OH SOY, OH SOY, OH BOY

The entire food industry has jumped on this bandwagon to promote the benefits of soy. We now have soy nuts, soy milk, soy burgers, soy chips, soy crackers and even soy candy bars. Women are consuming soy like it's the greatest deterrent of breast cancer ever available.

A debate looms, however, largely about the health value of non-fermented soy found in a great many processed foods mentioned above versus fermented soy considered to be a healthier alternative. We have looked to the Asian population and their incidence of breast cancer and have found it to be lower than in the United States. One difference between the two populations is the type of soy Asians are consuming, along with their high consumption of greens, garlic and tea.

"Soy has been correlated with low rates of breast cancer in Asian populations, but soy foods in Asia are made from minimally processed soybeans, or defatted, toasted soy flour, which is quite different from soy products consumed in the U.S.," said William G. Helferich, a professor of food science and human nutrition at the University of Illinois, Urbana. Much of their soy is also consumed in the form of miso, tempe and tofu. Highly-purified soy foods and soy supplements marketed in the United States may stimulate the growth of pre-existing estrogen-dependent breast tumors.

As Allan Spreen, M.D., advisor to the Health Science Institute in Baltimore Maryland says, *"When you take the basic components of the soybean, and then add to that the modern procedures of cultivation and mass production, you have a highly processed food of dubious nutritional value."*

Some studies have shown that soy has provided benefits by decreasing breast cancer risks. However, other studies have raised questions and dilemmas about the benefits versus the risks of soy as its use relates to breast cancer prevention.

The Chinese did not eat unfermented soybeans, as they did other legumes such as lentils, because the unfermented soybean contains large quantities of natural toxins or "anti-nutrients". These anti-nutrients are enzyme inhibitors that block the action of trypsin, an enzyme needed to digest protein. These anti-nutrients can produce gastric upset and reduce protein digestion.

In animal tests, high levels of trypsin inhibitors caused enlargement and pathological conditions of the pancreas, including cancer.

Other experts claim that although trypsin inhibitors may adversely affect the pancreas in animals, there is no solid evidence that they cause similar problems in humans. Even though trypsin inhibitors are found in the cabbage family and in beans, no one is suggesting that we not eat these highly nutritious foods. I believe it's a matter of consuming foods in moderation.

The Japanese, who eat 30 times as much soy as North Americans, have a lower incidence of cancers of the breast, uterus and prostate. But the Japanese and Asians in general, have much higher rates of other types of cancer, such as cancer of the esophagus, stomach, pancreas and liver.

It is the isoflavones in soy that are said to have a favorable effect on postmenopausal symptoms, including hot flashes and protection from osteoporosis. Quantification of discomfort from hot flashes is extremely subjective, however, and most studies show that there is very little difference in the amount of decreased discomfort experienced by those who were given soy versus those who were not given soy.

The FDA has claimed that isoflavones may work to "speed up" the proliferation of cancer cells that are dependent on estrogen for their growth. Other studies have found that soy stimulated potentially cancerous cell growth in pre-menopausal women. Still other studies have shown that soy consumption has had little effect on vasomotor symptoms such as night sweats, vaginal dryness and hot flashes.

The Solae Company is one of the world's largest soy producers, co-owned by Bunge Limited (an international agribusiness giant) and DuPont. They are submitting to the FDA a request to make the claim that soy helps prevent cancer. In light of what the FDA knows, plus claims already made about the potential side effects of soy, it will be worth watching and waiting to see the response from the FDA.

All of this conflicting, confusing information puts women in a quandary. We do know that soy phytoestrogens have an estrogenic effect of stimulating the growth of cancer cells in the laboratory. Several studies confirm this. Perhaps it would be wise, then, to consume soy, and preferably fermented soy products, in moderation while the jury is still out.

Even if we find out in the future, based on conclusive evidence, that soy may not stimulate the growth of cancer cells in the human breast, as always, balance and moderation is what we are trying to achieve.

COENZYME Q10 (CoQ10)

Coenzyme Q10 (ubiquinone) is used by the body as an antioxidant. An antioxidant protects cells from free radicals, which are highly reactive chemicals, often containing oxygen atoms. Free radicals are capable of damaging important cellular molecules such as DNA and lipids. In addition, the plasma level of CoQ10 has been used in studies as a measure of oxidative stress, a situation in which normal antioxidant levels are reduced. Some studies have suggested that CoQ10 stimulates the immune system and increases resistance to disease. This is why many researchers theorized that CoQ10 may be useful as an adjuvant therapy for cancer.

In 1993, after 35 years of clinical research on CoQ10, complete regression of tumors in two cases of breast cancer were reported. Three additional breast cancer patients also underwent a conventional protocol of therapy which included a daily oral dosage of 390 mg of vitamin CoQ10 over three to five years. Metastases in the liver of one patient "disappeared," and no signs of metastases were found elsewhere. Another patient, on a dosage of 390 mg of vitamin CoQ10, reported no signs of tumors, and the other patient showed no cancer or metastases. Although this research reflects a small number of cases, a good point to observe from this scientific data is the relationship of vitamin supplementation and its effects on treating and preventing cancer.

A more recent study indicated that women with breast cancer show a decrease of CoQ10 levels, and the later stage a cancer is in, the lower the amounts of CoQ10 present. We are learning so much more about the value of CoQ10. CoQ10 is used to help maintain heart health, promote healthy cholesterol levels, boost cellular energy and fight free-radical production. It is obvious that it is one of the nutrients we need the most.

ADD DIINDOLYLMETHANE (DIM) TO YOUR DIET

DIM is a plant compound called indole, which has been shown in many human and animal studies to help regulate and promote a more efficient metabolism of estrogen and to encourage an optimal ratio of estrogen metabolites. It is found in cruciferous vegetables such as broccoli, cabbage, cauliflower and brussel sprouts; these vegetables possess unique phytochemical constituents that are able to modify the metabolism of estrogen.

DIM also appears to suppress the growth of cancerous cells in the breast, prostate and cervix. To measure the ratio of good estrogen metabolites, a urine analysis 2/16 test can be done. The 2/16 ratio test measures your ratio of "good" 2-hydroxy-estrogen to "bad" 16a-hydroxy-estrogen. The same 2/16 ratio test that is recommended to women to determine their risk of breast cancer can also be used to help predict prostate cancer risk in men. It's available through Meridian Valley Laboratory (425.271.8689). Work with an integrative healthcare practitioner who is familiar with this test and its value. More information about this test can be found in the *Resource* section at the back of this book through the Tacoma Clinic.

Incorporating more cruciferous vegetables daily is a great way to increase the good estrogen ratio. Some women may need to take a DIM supplement (60 mg. 3 times daily) to get a good start to augment the intake of vegetables, particularly the women who are in a higher risk category for breast cancer.

Supplemental use of DIM provides the basis for nutritional support to enhance the beneficial action and safety of estrogen. An optimal "estrogen balance" has implications for cancer prevention and successful aging in both women and men.

Please don't wait until the pharmaceutical industry takes the natural form of DIM and molecularly changes it for patentable capabilities and aggressively markets it to the public. Mother Nature currently has it available for your taking. DIM is safe and will introduce you to a whole new world of healthy and tasty vegetables.

*S*tay informed and do not be lured by the attractive marketing that goes into fancy popular foods. Your health is at stake. Making good, healthy choices will determine the quality of your life throughout your lifetime. Remember, eating *"good"* fats, even butter and coconut oil in moderation, has its place. Contrary to popular belief, avoiding fats altogether or consuming a low fat diet can be detrimental to your health.

Last Nutritional Tip

Always read food labels and avoid, if possible, foods that contain the hydrogenated oils we discussed earlier. The purchase of fresh organic foods can help to avoid all the mystery in the labeling on regular food packages. With the use of e-commerce gaining momentum, it is now possible to have foods shipped from other parts of the country that are fresh and not processed. As an example, Seattle, Washington is a great place to purchase healthy, non-farmed salmon.

BIRTH CONTROL PILLS/ORAL CONTRACEPTIVES . . . NOT

Birth control pills, when first introduced to the marketplace, contained high levels of synthetic estrogen and progestin. Over the years, due to the devastating side effects of the Pill, lower dosages were developed in hopes of avoiding further death and illness. All the hoping in the world will not and cannot change the outcomes of the side effects of the lower dosage pills used today.

Birth control pills work by essentially putting the female body into a state of controlled menopause. The brain is fooled into thinking that the body is pregnant; therefore, a pregnancy cannot occur. It's always dangerous to fool Mother Nature, and we are seeing the results, some of which are not very pleasant.

It's interesting to observe that men in our culture are not expected to alter their sexuality through chemical treatments. They are not asked to suppress and subvert their normal reproductive functions. It is women who sacrifice their sexual integrity for birth control methods.

Oral contraceptives also have a potent carcinogenic effect. They raise a woman's chances of suffering from cervical cancer, liver tumors and breast cancer. They are linked to increased incidence of migraine headaches, vaginal infections, gallbladder disease, changes in vision, and a host of other clinical problems, including death. Oral contraceptive use also enhances the risk of contracting Chlamydia, a sexually transmitted disease, which is the leading cause of pelvic inflammatory disease (PID) in the U.S.

Approximately 10 million American women take oral contraceptives at any given time, but due to the negative side effects, one-third to one-half stop using them within a year.

Placing young adult women into a controlled *fooled* state with synthetic hormones like HRT has increased breast cancer and vascular events in women on the Pill. More specifically, the Pill can cause infertility, depression, high blood pressure, headaches, insulin resistance, high triglycerides, break-through bleeding, bloating, edema, rashes, dizziness, breast tenderness, and vision disturbances. Should we not look at the Pill more critically since the symptoms described above have become fairly common in young women today?

Even though they may be effective and convenient for women, the use of birth control pills comes at a price. Numerous studies report many health problems associated with their use, such as cardiovascular disease, breast cancer, uterine cancer and gall bladder disease. Research reports a 2.75-fold higher risk of ischemic stroke for oral contraceptive users compared with non-users. A meta-analysis of 16 trials focusing on this relationship found that the risks increase along with a low dose use of estrogens. What's interesting, however, is that other studies found that low dose usage of estrogens did not pose a risk.

In a study conducted in 2002, results indicated that even users of the "mini pill" have a 22 percent increase in breast cancer versus childless women who have not used oral contraceptives. Another study found that women using the pill were 2.7 times more likely to have lobular carcinoma of the breast than non-pill users. No difference in incidence of ductal carcinoma was found.

Despite the fact that we have documented studies that report the dangers of using oral contraceptives, and we are experiencing breast cancer, heart disease, stroke and other debilitating conditions in epidemic proportions, scientists are at it again. At the annual meeting of the American Society for Reproductive

Medicine in Philadelphia 2004, data extracted from the Women's Health Initiative study reported that the use of birth control pills is safe.

Well, ladies, you can figure this one out. The makers of these drugs just will not give up in trying to find a condition or medical need for their drugs. Though this confuses some women, more informed women know that this type of reporting has been going on since the 1960s with the marketing of HRT. Women must decide how much risk they are willing to take for a modern day convenience.

There are several more studies to which I can refer. However, the point has been made that these so-called benign birth control pills do, in fact, pose a real risk to women. An even more compelling point to draw attention to in this example is the arrogance with which the established medical community regards its scientific scrutiny.

This community believes that their scientific reporting is the *only* gold standard in the business. Yet, repeatedly we find that safety and effectiveness cannot be taken for granted, even when these scientists report their findings. Their philosophies about all women's healthcare issues work against the body's natural processes.

Remember, all these studies I've extrapolated as examples, come directly from established medical journals, yet those of us who purport safety and health from natural approaches are criticized without objective knowledge.

It is not popular to communicate the dangers of birth control pills to women today because their use has become so much a part of our social and behavioral fabric in the modern world. As unpopular as this might be, it is critically important to remind and inform women of the dangers of the Pill even though there are scientific studies to the contrary.

Again, the same mentality used to promote the use of HRT

in the early 1960s is what is being used to promote the use of birth control pills today. The true and devastating effects of birth control pills are coming back to haunt us as with HRT. Don't believe everything you are being told. There is no fooling Mother Nature, nor an informed woman.

No one is suggesting going back in time, but rather, women need to know the truth about birth control pills and the availability of other options that are safe and effective in order to make an informed decision. The operative word here is *safe*.

NATURAL FAMILY PLANNING...THE BILLINGS OVULATION METHOD (BOM), A HEALTHY ALTERNATIVE

Contrary to popular belief, there is a very safe and effective means of managing fertility without drugs, a means that women have been told for years is ineffective. The beauty of a natural approach to fertility is undeniable. First of all, it is safe and carries no harmful side effects from a health perspective. Secondly, it enables a woman to learn about her own body cycle, giving her deeper insight into her womanhood and the dignity of being a woman. Much of this attitude has been lost in the quest to become *"liberated"*.

This understanding is very useful throughout a women's lifetime, as she will quickly learn to detect the development of abnormalities. Thirdly, natural family planning engenders cooperation and respect between the woman and man and makes the responsibility for birth control a shared responsibility. Lastly, natural methods help the woman and man to develop love and concern for each other and for the child, thus enriching their relationship.

Some may consider this an old-fashioned approach. I like to think of it as a wise, safe, healthy, respectful and prudent approach. Once learned, the method can be applied to all variations throughout a woman's reproductive life:

- regular cycles
- irregular cycles
- anovular cycles
- effects of stress
- low fertility after childbirth or miscarriage
- while breastfeeding and weaning
- approaching menopause

The Billings Method provides a way to manage this important dimension, naturally and without harm of any kind. It recognizes fertility as a gift to be cherished, not as a condition which requires medication. The knowledge empowers women and lifts their status in the eyes of their husbands. It enhances communication in marriage, thereby strengthening the family bond.

Another natural method of fertility is **Fertility**_Care_™, which provides state-of-the-art, standardized instruction for achieving and avoiding pregnancy and for timing conception.

Its advantages are numerous. It is:

- highly effective and safe
- thoroughly researched
- inexpensive
- able to be used at any stage of a woman's reproductive life
- does not use harmful drug or devices
- respectful of natural biologic processes

This method has been found to be 99.5% effective in avoiding pregnancy. It has also been effective up to 40 percent of the time in helping women achieve pregnancy.

Natural Family Planning, whether you use BOM or **Fertility**_Care_™ is a versatile method that can be used in all stages of reproductive life. It is easy to learn, inexpensive, and is an extremely healthy alternative for those of you who choose to avoid riskier methods that increase the chances for illness and disease.

Both of these methods of managing fertility are based upon the changes in mucus secretions women experience during the month that cleverly indicate when a woman is fertile (ovulating). For more information about these natural approaches to fertility, visit the *Resource* section at the back of this book.

AVOID ANTIDEPRESSANTS

A recent study, conducted in 2003, reported that there is no association between anti-depressants and an increased risk for breast cancer. But there is more.

A second study in 2003 examined data from more than 930 women with invasive breast cancer and 510 women with *in situ* carcinoma and more than 1,200 who were cancer free.

Their findings reported that there was no connection between the use of antidepressants and an increased risk of breast cancer and that the relationship between duration of antidepressant use and incidences of breast cancer was inconsistent. What they did find, however, was an increased risk for invasive breast cancer if a woman took selective serotonin reuptake inhibitors (SSRI's) like Prozac, Paxil and Zoloft for at least three years.

Researchers concluded that the finding was insignificant, as "the demonstrated benefits of this class of drugs in treating depression probably outweigh the possible risk of breast cancer." *Probably outweighed the possible risk of breast cancer?* With such a horrific disease being reported in epidemic proportions, it's hard to believe that researchers would make such a nonchalant statement about risks versus benefits. This exact mindset is what started the slippery slope with the dangers of HRT 50 years ago. Everything appeared to be fine in the beginning; then ugly reports began showing up.

In another study, researchers found that heavy use of tricyclic antidepressants (TCA's) was shown to double the risk for breast cancer. Asendin, Anafranil, Norpramine, Petofrane, Rhotrimine, and Surmontil, were found to be genotoxic, meaning they are toxic to your DNA and may lead to mutations. Paxil, a popular SSRI, was also associated with an increased risk for breast cancer.

In 2000, the *American Journal of Epidemiology* found that women who use TCA's for more than two years may double their risk for breast cancer and that Paxil may also significantly increase a woman's risk of breast cancer. A sad commentary is that many of my clients have been prescribed Paxil for no reason other than to help them *"chill out"*. This is not a good clinical indicator for the use of a powerful drug that has potential risks.

For any woman currently using these drugs, I would suggest you consider an alternative. Work with a healthcare professional who will wean you from these drugs and explore the use of safer interventions.

An example of one of these alternatives, Tryptophan, is an important precursor to the brain chemical serotonin, which helps regulate mood. 100-200 mgs. of 5-Hydroxytryptophan (5-HTP), a close relative of tryptophan, can be used in divided doses along with 50-100 mg of vitamin B6 to ensure 5-HTP's conversion to serotonin.

Numerous double-blind studies have shown that 5-HTP has equal effectiveness compared to SSRIs such as Prozac, Paxil and Zoloft. The advantages range from being gentler and less expensive, to being associated with fewer and milder side effects.

Tryptophan is an amino acid (protein building block) that the body converts to serotonin, a neurotransmitter, that is frequently unbalanced in depressive individuals. Conventional antidepressants work to increase neurotransmitter levels by blocking their breakdown. According to Dr. Joseph Mercola, Director of the Optimal Wellness Center in Schaumburg, IL, it makes more sense to give the body more building blocks to make more of the serotonin.

Tryptophan works well with additional nutrients like folic acid and vitamin B6. Dr. Mercola recommends 3 mg of folic acid three times a day and Pyridoxal 5 phosphate (phosphorylated B6) 100-150 mg twice a day. The tryptophan dose is about 1500 mg, but can go to 3000 mg, usually taken at night. It is also helpful for insomnia.

Those who suffer from depression can also be protein deficient. Consuming more protein to get sufficient amounts of amino acids often improves depression without the use of supplements.

While the popularity of using drugs to alter brain chemistry continues to be a quick intervention, helping patients gain more control over their lives will actually produce even greater biochemical changes. One powerful technique is teaching individuals to be more optimistic. Depression can often be due to an underlying organic (chemical) or physiological cause. Addressing the underlying cause should be the primary therapy. Failure to do so will make any antidepressant therapy less successful.

Natural progesterone crème is also a very safe and effective intervention that will support the hormonal balance and deficiencies that cause depression, as was discussed in Chapter 3, Balancing Hormones…A safer and gentler approach.

Abortion and the Breast Cancer (ABC) Link

Although abortion is controversial, contentious, political, emotional and a subject of religious debate, I must address it from a health perspective that is often overlooked.

Charles B. Simone, M.D., is clinical director at the Simone Protective Cancer Institute in Lawrenceville, New Jersey and author of, *Breast Health: What You Need to Know.* He is also a medical oncologist, radiation oncologist and immunologist. He writes: *"When conception occurs, hormonal changes influence the breast. The milk duct network grows quickly to form other networks that will ultimately produce milk. During this period of tremendous growth and development, breast cells are undergoing great change and are immature or 'undifferentiated'; hence, they are more susceptible to carcinogens. But when a first full term pregnancy is completed, hormonal changes occur that permanently alter the breast network to greatly reduce the risk of outside carcinogen influence. When a termination occurs in the first trimester, there are no protective effects, and many of the rapidly dividing cells of the breast are left in transitional states....It is in these transitional states of high proliferation and undifferentiation that these cells can undergo transformation to cancer cells."*

Therefore, if a woman who has gone through some weeks or months of a normal pregnancy chooses abortion, she is left with more of these cancer-vulnerable cells in her breasts than were there before she got pregnant, raising her risk of breast cancer later in life. Is this discussed during a consult prior to a woman making her final decision about abortion? We would like to think so.

A full term pregnancy after a woman has had an abortion can help reduce her chances for developing the disease later in life. A full term pregnancy enables a woman to develop cancer-resistant tissue. This is why women who have more children have a lower lifetime risk for breast cancer.

Another compelling piece of information reported by Janet Daling from a research study is that when young women over the age of 18 (with a known family history of breast cancer) had an abortion, their risk of disease increased substantially. All 12 women in this study with this history were diagnosed with breast cancer by the age of 45.

Let me explain the estrogen connection, too. Estrogen, as we have learned in earlier chapters, is a powerful and necessary hormone. It is the chemical messenger that turns a young girl's body, during puberty, into a woman's body. There is a cast of estrogens responsible for this miraculous process that stimulates the growth of breasts and other female tissues.

In fact, the actions of most known risk factors for breast cancer are attributable to some form of estrogen overexposure, hence the HRT debacle. In a normal pregnancy, the mother's ovaries begin producing extra estrogen within a few days after conception. The level of estrogen in her blood rises some 2,000 percent by the end of the first trimester, to a level more than six times higher than it ever gets in the non-pregnant state. *"The only mechanism that protects breast tissue from overexposure to estrogen, and matures the tissue into cancer-resistant, milk-producing tissue, is a process known as differentiation that begins at 32 weeks of pregnancy. If a woman has an abortion, or a pre-term birth before 32 weeks of gestation, her breast-cancer risk may increase. Most first-trimester miscarriages, however, have not been linked to increased cancer risk because there is no estrogen overexposure."*, says Karen Malec, president of the Coalition on Abortion/Breast Cancer. The culprits here are the undifferentiated cells in the breasts, stimulated by estrogen to proliferate, so that there will be enough milk-producing tissue to feed the baby after birth. Only the undifferentiated cells are vulnerable to carcinogens, and can ultimately grow into cancer cells.

Importantly, during the last 8 weeks of pregnancy, other hormones differentiate these cells into milk-producing cells. In the process, the growth potential and cancer-forming potential of these cells is turned off. That is why a full-term pregnancy lowers the risk of breast cancer later in life.

In contrast, most pregnancies which abort spontaneously (miscarriages) do not generate normal quantities of estrogen. Thus, most miscarriages (at least 1st trimester miscarriages) do not raise breast cancer risk.

It is widely known that women who start having children at a younger age lower their risk of getting breast cancer later in life. The sooner the breasts become fully mature for the purpose of milk production, the less likely the presence of abnormal, potentially cancer-forming cells from accumulated carcinogenic insults.

Many medical experts today agree that the best way women can reduce their risk of breast cancer is to have an early (before age 24) first full term pregnancy (FFTP), to bear more children, and to breastfeed for a longer duration. It's quite clear that abortion causes women to change their child bearing patterns.

Scientists at Harvard and Oxford have reported that decreased childbearing and breastfeeding account for at least 50 percent of the breast cancer cases in the developed world. Yet, researchers from the National Cancer Institute (NCI), Center of Disease Control (CDC) and the American Cancer Society (ACS) appear to be in denial about the physiological changes in a woman's breasts during pregnancy and abortion.

In spite of the dangers of abortion to women's health, the issue has been more politicized (a women's right to her own body) and there have been efforts to squelch the truth. Is this politics and economics trumping science again?

There is a common thread that runs throughout the history of women's health issues that has not been fully disclosed. The first American study published found that a "first trimester abortion before first full term pregnancy, whether spontaneous (miscarriage) or induced, was associated with a 2.4 fold increase in breast cancer risk."

Thirty-eight epidemiological studies exploring an independent link with breast cancer and abortion have been published. Of these, 29 reported increased risk.

These are just a few cited examples of research that have not been shared with the public at large. Where are all the major newspaper and magazine publishers on this issue? Although some publications have provided fair coverage of this issue, i.e., *WorldNetDaily*, *Report News Magazine*, *Cybercast News Service*, *Chicago Tribune*, the *Indianapolis Star* and the *National Catholic Register*, this group pales in comparison to the small amount of coverage by the media at large.

Why might this information have been carefully buried? It could be due to fear of disrupting the current operations of very large profitable organizations and institutions.

In 2000, a former editor of the Journal of the American Medical Association *JAMA*, George Lundberg, M.D., told an interviewer that abortion, like tobacco, is one of the *"sensitive issues"* that has been on the American Medical Association (AMA's) *"don't touch list"* for many years.

As of 2001, the AMA did not have a policy about informing women about the abortion/breast cancer ABC research.

If you visit the AMA's website today, this is what you will see: *The issue of support of or opposition to abortion is a matter for members of the AMA to decide individually, based on personal values or beliefs. The AMA will take no action which may be construed as an attempt to alter or influence the personal views of individual physicians regarding abortion procedures.*

So in other words, the AMA will not take a clinical stand on a surgical procedure that has been reported in several scientific journals as being a contributing factor to the increased risk of breast cancer.

On the other hand, if AMA members choose natural

methods of healing, some of which have been discussed in previous chapters, based upon their personal values or beliefs, methods that are not acceptable practices within the halls of conventional medicine, the AMA is ready to drag them before their medical boards, discipline them, and accuse them of practicing voo-doo medicine. Is there a double-standard here?

The AMA's stance on this issue should send up red flags everywhere that not only warn women of the dangers of abortion, but also disclose the half-truths and deception around this issue.

At the Miami Breast Cancer Conference in March 2000, Dan Osman M.D., conference director, was asked if he knew there was a link between abortion and breast cancer. He said *"yes"* and when asked why there couldn't be a presentation about it at the meeting he said it was "too political".

There are more doctors today who are becoming more informed and are being straightforward about research findings and breast cancer risk. Some doctors who were initially skeptical have started obtaining a complete reproductive history on their patients and have found that many cases of breast cancer in young women are associated with an abortion history.

Joel Brind, Ph.D., is the founder and president of the Breast Cancer Prevention Institute and is a professor of biology and endocrinology at City University of New York's Baruch College. Dr. Brind concluded from a report that *"Abortion can explain the entire rise in breast cancer since the mid 1980s. It's not just because of the rise in women young enough to have had an abortion, it's also that the absolute numbers of increased cases fall within the range of numbers we predicted in our 1996 meta-analysis."*

Some of the latest scientific findings in the United Kingdom have also been disturbing, particularly since the incidence of breast cancer in this region is growing at the same time that access to treatment is being delayed.

A London-based researcher, Patrick Carroll, presented a report to the *British Journal of Cancer* showing that legal induced abortion - especially before first full term pregnancy – is the "best predictor of English breast cancer trends." Biologic evidence states that abortions before first time full pregnancy are highly carcinogenic. Carroll used British government statistics for his data - not women's interviews (often incomplete) and not computerized medical records. This data is superior to that of some nations, including the U.S., as it captures a record of nearly every breast cancer and abortion.

Although Carroll has reported these research findings extracted from London's very own governmental statistics, he is being ignored by London Health Officials. The longer these statistics are ignored, the faster incidence of breast cancer mortality rates will rise.

It's almost shameful the way health and medical information is being withheld about the link between abortion and breast cancer. Women have the exclusive right to be their own decision makers when it comes to their own healthcare concerns. Sorting out the science and the truth on abortion is critical in order for women to understand the health implications and to make an informed decision.

Politics must not and should not prohibit open discussion and evaluation of the scientific literature. Every woman has the right to know!

"If you want the rainbow,
you gotta put up with the rain."
—Dolly Parton

6

OSTEOPOROSIS...A PERSONAL STORY

I AM COMPELLED TO BEGIN this chapter with a personal story involving my mother because there is a powerful message to be learned from her experience.

My mother was diagnosed with severe osteoporosis at the age of 74. She had lost two inches in height; her doctor said she had never seen such poor bones in all her years of practicing medicine. The doctor was practically in a panic because her own father had suffered severe osteoporosis over the years and had lost four inches in height by the age of 62. He had become nearly crippled over a very short period of time due to the bone loss.

She immediately recommended Fosamax as the first means of intervention, for fear my mother would break a bone sometime soon. It was not an issue of *"if"*, but *"when"* Mom would break a bone. This condition, which causes weak, brittle bones, is one of the main culprits in hip fractures, so I thoroughly understood her concern.

This practicing pattern of medical treatment for osteoporosis is typical in medical circles today, but that does not necessarily make it the best line of intervention, as you will soon find out, because it is only treating the symptoms.

Having followed and studied the writings and research of Dr.

Lee and his colleagues for years, I knew this was not the route I wanted my mother to pursue. A combination of reviewing scientific literature, my intuition and experience, and my mother's willingness to follow Lee's recommendations brought about an incredible outcome that all women need to hear about.

Our next step was to meet with Mom's physician and explain to her why we would choose another intervention that included a multiple lifestyle approach versus the drug route. The physician was very concerned because she feared mom would break a bone before she would experience improvement in her bone status. We agreed that we would follow our plan of action for eighteen months and re-measure her bone density at that time. The doctor was not pleased with our plan, but nonetheless, we proceeded.

I share this with you, because it is important and highly recommended to work with your healthcare professionals and share the research with them, research that they rarely see. As I mentioned in earlier chapters, physicians are only exposed to literature the pharmaceutical companies produce about their drugs. Therefore, they have very little knowledge, if any, about lifestyle changes and more natural approaches to healing conditions and illness.

Rather than subject Mom to the serious side effects of a bisphosphonate such as Fosamax, (side effects like ulceration of the esophagus, vision problems, ulcers, joint pain, brittle bones, nausea, headaches, damage to the gastric lining, and liver damage), we chose to address this condition through exercise, good eating, dietary supplements and the use of natural progesterone crème, a treatment approach that is well documented in the scientific literature.

As a side note, biphosphonate drugs are toxic poisons that contain the same type of chemicals that are used to remove soap scum from your bathtub. It should be no surprise that serious side effects occur.

Mom has always been an active woman who walks three miles per day, consumes a variety of foods in moderation, is not overweight and has taken multi-vitamins since she was forty years old.

She continued her walking regime and increased her consumption of green vegetables such as spinach, cabbage, kale and other greens. We added a combination mineral supplement that included calcium, magnesium, boron and vitamin D. She also began using a two-ounce tube of natural progesterone crème every month. It was just a little tweaking in her current lifestyle that made all the difference.

After eighteen months on this regimen, she had another bone density test. Her physician was shocked when she received the results. Her left femoral changed from -3.09 to -2.1 and her L2 and L4 region changed from -.43 to +.6. She actually grew bone and was no longer classified as osteoporotic! The improvement was dramatic. This intervention enabled Mom to continue living her life as usual with a few minor adjustments and the results were phenomenal.

She has continued with this lifestyle regime ever since, and I am happy to report that she just turned 81 this year. I am not only proud of her, but extremely happy that we have been able to manage this condition as a result of her commitment and desire to work at healing herself. Lee's program was a success, just as he had recommended. Sure we could have taken the route of a pharmaceutical drug. Some studies show that Fosamax does slightly slow bone loss and has been known to modestly increase bone mass. We achieved excellent results by avoiding the side affects that so often accompany the use of powerful drugs. The whole idea behind correcting this condition is to grow bone in order to decrease the risk of bone breakage.

The results of using natural progesterone crème are often

dramatic in older women with serious bone loss, yet when do you ever hear of a physician making this recommendation?

Progesterone, *not* synthetic progestin, has been shown in many examples to increase bone mass and density. Jerilynn Prior, M.D. at the University of British Columbia in Vancouver, British Columbia, Canada, reported that osteoporosis developed in women who were progesterone deficient and estrogen dominant. Modest bone benefit resulted from the use of progestin (the synthetic progesterone), but to a lesser degree than the benefits from natural progesterone.

Mark Helfand Ph.D., a member of a National Institutes of Health (NIH) consensus panel, reported this in the Washington Post, *"Even people who agree that osteoporosis is a serious health problem can still say it is being hyped. Most of what you could do to prevent osteoporosis later in life has nothing to do with getting a test or taking a drug."*

Much of the literature addressing osteoporosis that is being promoted by the media today is often misleading, inaccurate, and supportive of the drug industry in disguise. Despite contradictory evidence published in the medical journals, conventional wisdom has convinced doctors and patients alike that osteoporosis has reached epidemic proportions. They now believe that without immediate intervention, including yearly diagnostic screenings and prescription drugs, a woman is bound to suffer from fractures.

Stanford University researchers reported that as of 2003, there were an estimated 3.6 million people who had been diagnosed with osteoporosis, compared with half a million in 1994. The number of doctor visits had increased from 1.3 million in 1994 to 6.3 million in 2003. These increases coincided with the introduction of supposedly bone-protecting drugs such as Fosamax, Evista and Actonel. Could this all be due to masterful marketing on the part of the drug companies?

These drugs, however, continue to lose popularity due to the recent studies reporting direct links to heart problems, breast cancer and other risk factors. Randall Stafford, who led the study, commented, "We hope to catch it early enough to treat it early enough to prevent fractures."

Do you ever wonder why it is taking the medical establishment so long to embrace prevention? Preventive-minded practitioners have been espousing this for years.

So there you have it. Another condition classified as a disease that is not a disease can be prevented. Unfortunately, drug intervention is the first line of defense in medical circles rather than teaching and informing women that lifestyle behaviors with nutrition, exercise and supplements is safer and more effective. The medical institutions should be placing the majority of their resources in teaching young girls and women how to *"prevent"* this condition from occurring in the first place.

The evidence is in. Drugs are *not* the answer for osteoporosis. They cause more risks than benefits. It's wise always to evaluate the risk/benefit ratio when contemplating any type of drug regime. I have yet to see a greater benefit with drug use when it comes to treating chronic illnesses and conditions with the exception of insulin for diabetes.

Bone Up on the Facts

"Countries with the highest rates of osteoporosis, such as the United States, England, and Sweden, also consume the most milk. China and Japan, where people eat much less protein and dairy food, have low rates of osteoporosis." Is there something wrong with this picture?

The world of institutional medicine has done a great job in promoting myths and half-truths to women about osteoporosis. Women have been taught for the past 20 years that osteoporosis is a calcium deficiency disease, an estrogen deficiency disease and a menopausal disease, all of which are not true.

Osteoporosis literally means porous bone. It is the decalcification and weakening of bones. Bone is living tissue and continues to break down and rebuild throughout a life time. As a result of bone being living tissue, it needs nutrients like any living organism. However, the lack of calcium in the diet is not the only nutrient necessary to grow strong bones. There are a variety of other factors that effect bone mass that include magnesium, vitamin D, other minerals, hormones, lifestyle and other dietary considerations.

BONE UP ON GREENS AND SUPPLEMENTS

The best source of calcium is from the earth's soil. Broad-leafed vegetables provide a rich source of calcium. Phosphorus, magnesium and zinc follow as important minerals, too.

Phosphorus supplementation, however, is not necessary because the American diet consists of too many carbonated beverages and red meat. And when too much phosphorus is consumed, it can actually lead to bone loss.

Magnesium helps to increase calcium absorption and is necessary. Bone building supplements contain 2:1 calcium: magnesium ratio. A good place to start is consuming at least 300-500 mg/day. As a result of our modern food-growing processes, we are robbed of magnesium and most nutrients due to our depleted soils. We can find this rich mineral in vegetables, whole grains, nuts and seeds. Other robbers of calcium excretion are salt, sugar, and protein. Zinc, boron, and manganese (found in whole unprocessed foods) are essential, too.

VITAMINS:

Vitamin A is important for synthesis of connective tissue and for the composition of cartilage and bone. Most multivitamins contain about 5,000 IU of vitamin A recommended daily.

Beta-carotene, when consumed in foods, is readily converted to vitamin A in the body.

Vitamin B6 (pyridoxine), about 50-100 mgs. twice/day, is a helper in the production of progesterone.

Vitamin C, about 2,000-3,000 mgs. throughout the day is essential for the synthesis and repair of all collagen, cartilage and bone.

Vitamin D, comes from sunshine. It helps to convert the minerals into bone, enhances calcium absorption and plays an important role in the health of bones overall. Consuming 2,000-4,000 IU of vitamin D has been found to be very effective in protecting against a host of many conditions and illnesses.

A study conducted at Mount Sinai Hospital in Toronto provided 4,000 IU of vitamin D3 daily to men and women for two to five months. The study found no evidence of liver toxicity or calcium overload. Other researchers found that the FDA's previous "safe upper limit" of vitamin D (2000 IU daily) is actually too low by at least 5-fold. They also found that up to 10,000 IU of vitamin D daily appears safe.

Don't believe the conventional wisdom that an antacid is good defense against poor bones. In reality, antacids are not a very good source of calcium. They contain calcium carbonate, which is not absorbed as well as calcium citrate. Antacids also reduce gastric acidity, which reduces nutrient absorption overall. Additionally, medications such as antacids reduce our body's ability to absorb calcium.

Be aware also of the effects of salt. The hidden salts in processed foods are a major problem. Increased salt causes the kidneys to remove increased amounts of calcium from the blood and deposit it in the urine. As more calcium leaves the body, the bones become weaker.

Got Milk?...Hope not

The popular tag line **"Got Milk?"** is seen in hundreds of magazines and on billboards across the U.S. using Hollywood stars painted with milk mustaches. Using attractive stars has become popular to encourage consumers to increase their consumption of milk as a means of consuming more calcium in their diet. This marketing effort has been quite beneficial for the dairy industry. However, now that the numbers are in, the results are dismal, and the incidence of osteoporosis continues to grow in this country.

*L*et's apply a little logic and common sense to this milk agenda. A better choice for a calcium-rich diet is one rich in leafy vegetables, whole wheat, legumes, sesame seeds and brown rice.

Why then are we depending on the cows to consume those leafy greens and pass them on to us through the milk process, when we can get them directly from the ground ourselves through plants? Besides, one cup of leafy vegetables contains the same amount of calcium as one cup of milk.

Furthermore, most cows are fed a grain diet dosed with high levels of antibiotics and other drugs in order to fatten them up for greater milk production. Where do you think all these drugs go after they have passed through the cow's digestive system? Yes, that's right, to you and me, in the milk.

Heating milk to the high temperatures required for pasteurization destroys all the vital elements of the milk. To top this off, another part of the process is adding fortified vitamins (lost through pasteurization) back into the milk.

The *American Journal of Public Health* published a study in 1997 that studied 77,761 women, ages 34-59, and found no evidence that higher intake of cow's milk reduced fracture incidence. In fact, the opposite was found. Women who drank two or more glasses of milk daily actually had a significantly higher risk of bone fracture when compared to women who drank less than one glass of milk per week.

This is quite interesting, since Americans consume the greatest amount of calcium and have the highest incidence of osteoporosis. Could it be that cow's milk is *not* what it is mooed up to be? Now, if you have access to raw, unpasteurized milk, this is another story.

*W*omen are consuming plenty of calcium, and it is necessary for bone growth, but... it's other minerals, hormonal balance and lifestyle factors that provide the greatest benefit to bone growth.

Bone contains numerous alkaline minerals, including calcium, magnesium, and potassium. When our bodies become overly acidic from diet, stress, and lifestyle, these alkaline minerals leach from our bones to buffer the high acidity. Yet, even as bone is constantly being broken down, it's also constantly being rebuilt.

When our bodies begin to produce less progesterone and estrogen, our bones start to die very quickly. Estrogen controls osteoclast activity that dissolves the old bone and leaves room for new bone formation. Progesterone controls osteoblastic activity that produces or builds this new bone. As a result of this natural process, it is evident that a *balance* of hormones is what is necessary to avoid bone loss.

A Case for Natural Progesterone and Bones

Dr. Prior found that women developed osteoporosis when their estrogen levels were high. They had also stopped menstruating, which meant their progesterone levels had dropped. She found that it was the lack of progesterone that caused osteo porosis. Prior also showed evidence that osteoblasts (cells that form new bone) have progesterone receptors.

Dr. Lee found, after reviewing the medical charts of his patients, that those who were treated with natural progesterone only, along with a good diet, supplements and exercise had experienced a reversal in their osteoporosis. Progesterone stimulates the osteoblasts to make new bone.

Exercise, Exercise, Exercise

A recent published study indicates that exercise is more important than calcium intake in developing strong bones in girls and young women.

Researchers at Penn State University and Johns Hopkins University found that even among girls whose calcium intake was far below the recommended daily allowance, calcium did not significantly affect bone strength. Tom Lloyd, Ph.D., professor of health evaluation sciences at Penn State's College of Medicine at the Milton S. Hershey Medical Center, noted, however, that when the girls were asked about their exercise habits, the data showed a strong correlation between exercise and bone strength.

Studies have shown that women build most of their bone mass in their early and mid-teens. Bone mass then slowly erodes as women age. Building good bone mass in adolescence, then, is thought to be the best way to prevent osteoporosis in old age. Teach your children well and introduce them to healthy eating and other good lifestyle habits early on.

John Patnott, Ph.D., professor of kinesiology at Hope College in Holland, Mich., said he was not surprised by the findings. "Bones are very similar to muscles; you have to use them to develop strength," Patnott said. "I think that calcium in the diet is very important, but calcium by itself won't accomplish what is necessary without bone stress." So, if you want strong bones, exercise daily for at least thirty minutes.

Include weight-bearing exercises such as walking and weight lifting into a daily routine. This kind of activity has been shown to generate electrical current in bone that will stimulate growth. Such exercises improve bone strength and balance too. Stretching and strengthening exercises are as important to increasing bone strength as the consumption of raw/uncooked vegetables such as broccoli, spinach, kale, collards, dandelion greens, sprouts, seeds and nuts.

Try to eat red meat in moderation and organic meats, if possible, which come from grass fed animals. Finally, consume a good supplement that contains all the necessary minerals that help to protect and build bone. It's this whole package that keeps bones growing. Good bone enhancing supplements are available from the vitamin companies listed in *Resources* at the back of the book.

Claims of increased calcium, new drugs and HRT can be put to rest when you learn the truth behind the body's natural physiological processes. Surgeon General Richard Carmona agrees. Carmona beleives the focus must be on preventing thinning bones, not on medication.

IF YOU ARE DIAGNOSED WITH OSTEOPOROSIS

We know that this condition, when left untreated, can leave some devastating damage in its path. This is why preventing osteoporosis from occurring in the first place is the goal. However, if you are one of the unfortunate women who has been diagnosed with osteoporosis and are too impatient to slowly grow bone using my mother's approach, there is another option that can help to accelerate healing and bone growth.

Robert O. Becker, M.D., a pioneering scientist and orthopedic surgeon, has done a great deal of research in the area of electromagnet therapy (EMT). This therapy enhances overall cellular functions and assists the body to heal itself.

Retired now, Dr. Becker pioneered laboratory research in the field of regeneration of bone and muscle after injuries. He experimented with weak electrical currents while working at the Veterans Hospital in Syracuse and as Professor of Medicine at New York University's Upstate Medical Center.

Dr. Becker began much of his research in the 1960s, showing that electric current could stimulate the healing process in broken bones. EMT works by increasing the bioelectric energy of your body to create balance. When this balance occurs, energy is increased; this, in turn, stimulates healing.

Though osteoporosis is different than a bone fracture, EMT can help to slow down bone loss while you are incorporating other lifestyle behaviors such as exercise, mineral supplementation, improved nutrition and hormone balance.

Interest in EMT is gaining steam today. The FDA has approved EMT for the use of bone fractures that are unable to heal; EMT is also being used to fuse spinal vertebrae in people with chronic back pain. Some of the research is being combined with the use of magnets regarding negative and positive fields.

BONE DENSITY TESTS

It is a good idea to establish a baseline of bone density, so it can be tracked over time. There are a couple of ways to measure bone density. Dual energy X-ray absorptiometry (DEXA) usually takes measurements from both the hip and lumbar spine area. This test exposes people to less radiation than other X-ray techniques.

A urine test such as OsteoCheck or Osteomark-NTX

measures and keeps track of bone loss. This type of testing provides faster feedback than a DEXA test. Please remember these tests are diagnostic tools and should be repeated if there is any question about the results, especially if medications are recommended.

You need not fear osteoporosis any longer, now that you know how to prevent it. And even if you got a late start in learning about this condition, all of the recommendations discussed earlier can make a remarkable difference and can even reverse osteoporosis.

"Be who you are and say what you feel, because those who mind don't matter, and those that matter don't mind."
—Dr. Seuss

THE HEART OF THE MATTER
IS REVEALING

THE WOMEN AND HEART DISEASE fact sheet compiled by The National Coalition for Women with Heart Disease reports some of the following statistics:

- Heart disease is the leading cause of death of American women and kills 32 percent of them.
- 43 percent of deaths in American women, or nearly 500,000, are caused by cardiovascular disease (heart disease and stroke) each year.
- 267,000 women die each year from heart attacks, which kill six times as many women as breast cancer.
- 31,837 women die each year of congestive heart failure, or 62.6 percent of all heart failure deaths.
- 435,000 American women have heart attacks each year; 83,000 are under age 65 and 9,000 are under age 45. Their average age is 70.4.
- 13 percent of women age 45 and over have had a heart attack.

- Women with diabetes are two to three times more likely to have heart attacks.
- High blood pressure is more common in women taking oral contraceptives, especially in obese women.
- More women than men die of heart disease each year, yet women receive only:
  - 33 percent of angioplasties, stents and bypass surgeries,
  - 28 percent of implantable defibrillators and 36 percent of open-heart surgeries.
- Women comprise only 25 percent of participants in all heart-related research studies.

On top of this, the biggest and most shocking data extracted from the Women's Health Initiative (WHI) study, after it had been stopped dead in its tracks in 2002, revealed that hormone users had a 24 percent increase in heart disease risk. Some critics contend that there was only one year in all the heart data where there was a statistical increase, but evidently it was high enough to have frightened many women.

In 1998, the Heart and Estrogen/Progestin Replacement Study (HERS) reported an increased risk of heart attack soon after the start of hormone therapy. After one year, the women receiving hormone replacement therapy were more likely to have heart attacks or die from heart disease than the placebo group. After two years, this difference disappeared. During the 4th and 5th years, the women who used hormone replacement therapy had fewer heart attacks and deaths from heart disease than those who took a placebo. It is possible that hormone replacement therapy may increase your risk of heart disease initially, but may later become more effective in preventing heart disease. But who is willing to take this risk?

Prior to halting the WHI study, there was ample evidence

reported from other scientific studies stating the increased risks and dangers of synthetic hormones. We have learned that post-menopausal women have an increased risk of cardiovascular disease, which is now the leading cause of death in women. Hormone replacement therapy (synthetic hormones) has been shown to result in an increase in strokes in large prospective clinical trials.

One thing we know for sure; synthetic hormones *do not* protect the heart. Could this be why the statistics are so disturbing? Why would women agree to the use of synthetic hormones and place themselves at risk for coronary heart disease (CHD) and/or death knowing that this disease can be treated and/or reversed by diet and lifestyle behaviors?

This is a very compelling argument. Only physicians who claim they know a woman's body better than she knows it herself prescribe this treatment. How can logic such as this be called "good medicine"?

What I find so insidious is: if indeed we have determined increased risks with the use of synthetic hormones, then what type of scientific validity did we have prior to this information that established a cultural norm (HRT for all menopausal women) in creating practice patterns in medicine?

To add insult to injury, every woman, whether pre- or post-menopausal, had been prescribed the same dosage of these synthetic hormones. This is an example of why cookbook medicine is a failure.

PROGESTERONE...NOT PROGESTIN

The big question is WHY? Researchers at Oregon Regional Primate Research Center conducted a study that reported natural progesterone, not the synthetic progestin found in Provera, may help prevent heart attacks. It was also reported that Provera may increase the risk of heart attacks. There have been other researchers, too, who for some time have suspected that Provera's risks outweigh the benefits.

London's National Heart and Lung Institute conducted a study that revealed the beneficial effects natural progesterone had on reducing platelet aggregation through its ability to enhance endothelium-derived relaxing factor (nitric oxide).

Based upon the results of these studies, scientists have determined that progestin causes a major threat to a woman's health. Kent Hermsmeyer, Ph.D., one of the researchers at the Oregon Regional Primate Research Center states, "*The big surprise is that [Provera] poses such a huge risk. This is really a dangerous drug.*" Dr. J. Koudy Williams, a scientist from Wake Forest University, who conducted his research on monkeys, states that "*Provera is worse than no treatment at all.*"

Progestins interfere with vascularization, blood clotting, how cholesterol is metabolized by the endothelial cells lining the heart, and the calcium exchange that controls the firing in the heart muscle. Progestins block estrogen receptors, which change how our arteries dilate and respond to stimuli.

Progesterone also blocks estrogen but it does so in a natural physiological pattern. This is the way the body intended it to be because it is the hormone the body produces. Progestins are drugs which disrupt the entire electrical configuration of the heart.

Another study has gone awry because of incorrect conclusions and assumptions. "*Possible Peril Found in Menopause Cream*" is the title of the article. Use of Prometrium, an oral progesterone at 200 mg daily doses, was compared to the use of natural progesterone crème (ProGest) of 40 mg daily doses. The researchers' concern is that the oral micronized progesterone, Prometrium, was absorbed the same way as the natural progesterone, therefore, placing women at risk who purchase this crème over the counter.

Researchers also reported that the use of natural progesterone crème without medical supervision from a doctor was dangerous because of the risks of coronary artery disease, stroke, thrombosis and breast cancer. This makes absolutely no sense. Evidently, these researchers still do not understand the difference between progestins, which *do* increase the risks of coronary artery disease, stroke, thrombosis and breast cancer and natural progesterone crème. Furthermore, it appears as though their biggest concern is that women are using interventions without their professional assistance.

*H*mmm, seems like we have heard and seen this reaction before. This could be one more step toward regulating natural progesterone unless informed women in this country stand up to be heard.

Scientists' reactions to this study is another way of telling women they are not capable of making their own personal health care decisions. Frankly, more informed women today are doing much better without the recommendations from their physicians regarding the hormone argument. The statistics speak for themselves.

The medical community apparently cannot (or will not) grasp the physiology of the human body and the production of progesterone. In their studies, they are still using oral forms of progesterone (or progestin in most cases), which require them to prescribe amounts beyond what the body produces. Therein lies the problem.

If only Dr. Lee were still alive today to repeat one more time the crystal clear difference between synthetic progestins and natural progesterone. As he has questioned numerous times in the past:

- Why do fertility doctors always use progesterone and not progestins?
- Why do progestins cause birth defects, while progesterone is essential for a viable and healthy pregnancy?
- Why don't synthetic progestins show up in blood and saliva tests of progesterone levels? (In other words, why doesn't taking a progestin raise progesterone levels in the body?)
- Pregnant women are making 300 mg of progesterone daily in the last trimester. Why don't they have higher rates of breast cancer, as do women who use progestins? [In fact, women who have never been pregnant have a significantly increased risk of breast cancer.]
- Why doesn't natural progesterone cause the side effects listed for medroxyprogesterone acetate (Provera), the most commonly used synthetic progestin for HRT?

Recently, another study was conducted on the use of natural progesterone crème that would have delighted Lee. Thirty postmenopausal women received 20 mg. of natural progesterone crème daily for four weeks to assess relief of menopausal symptoms. Unlike the adverse effects from the use of Premarin and Provera, the study showed no harmful effects from the use of the crème.

Women who have been using natural progesterone creme for the relief of hot flashes, sleeplessness and mood swings should feel vindicated from the results of this study. As more studies of this type are conducted, I feel confident more women will embrace more natural approaches to protecting themselves from debilitating conditions, illness and disease.

These are just a few examples of multiple studies that have reported the risks of synthetic hormones as related to heart disease, yet several doctors and researchers are still convinced that they offer more benefit than risk. This is even more of a reason why women need to do their own reading and research and look outside of conventional medicine's mindset for safe and long term solutions.

Evidently, this has been a strong enough argument for informed women to have abandoned their synthetic hormones, but this is not and was not the research that encouraged women to take personal health matters into their own hands.

The relentless hours of research and book writing by Lee, and his commitment to lecture across the world, have opened the eyes of not only women, but of many scientists and researchers, as well. We are just beginning to see and understand why the value of using bio-identical hormones is a much safer and recommended approach for balancing hormones than use of the synthetic form that directly increases the risk of disease.

Informed women who have been using natural progesterone crème properly with positive results are having to work very hard to withstand the verbal abuse and intimidation from physicians and institutions. No woman to date has experienced death or increased risk to disease due to the use of natural progesterone crème, yet the critics are out in full force to discredit its use.

The medical community's behavior reminds me of an experiment that was conducted to capture monkeys. A nut was placed inside a narrow-mouthed jar where the monkey could find it. Once the monkey saw the treat, it reached into the jar to grab it, but was unable to remove its hand without letting go of the treat. As a result of holding on to the treat, the monkey was captured. Holding on to the treat was far more important than freedom.

The medical community clings to a theory (like the monkey and its treat) that has been scientifically validated as risky in order to maintain its hunger for control and power. It's just more important to be "right" than to do the right thing. In this case, however, women are being placed at risk and are suffering needlessly. The goal in medicine should be to assist and heal, not to be self-righteous and controlling.

ESTROGEN IS DANGEROUS WHEN NOT USED PROPERLY

Estrogen's direct link to cardiovascular disease has also been reported in studies. Another part of the WHI study found that estrogen-alone hormone therapy had no effect on coronary heart disease risk but increased the risk of stroke for post-menopausal women. The study also found that estrogen-alone therapy significantly increased the risk of deep vein thrombosis, but had no significant effect on the risk of breast or colorectal cancer. It also reduced the risk of hip and other fractures.

This portion of the study (estrogen-alone) was halted at the end of February 2004 because the hormone increased the risk of stroke and did not reduce the risk of coronary heart disease, which was a key question in the trial. The study was to have ended in March 2005.

*I*nitial findings appear in the April 14 issue of *The Journal of the American Medical Association.* "The results make clear that hormone therapy does not protect women against coronary heart disease and increases their risk for stroke," said Dr. Jacques Rossouw, WHI Project Officer at the National Heart, Lung and Blood Institute (NHLBI). "This may be especially true for older women, such as those aged 60 and older in this study."

"These findings confirm that estrogen-alone therapy should not be used to prevent chronic disease," said NHLBI Acting

Director Dr. Barbara Alving. "We believe the findings support current FDA recommendations that hormone therapy only be used to treat menopausal symptoms and that it be used at the smallest effective dose for the shortest possible time." Of course, we, the informed, also have learned that using synthetic hormone therapy to treat menopausal symptoms in any case, is not safe. They just can't let go of their synthetic hormones.

Brainwashing is the only way to describe how our medical professionals have been trained. The notion that synthetic estrogen could still be used for menopausal symptoms for a short time is like playing Russian roulette. Are you willing to take that risk, knowing that there are alternatives that are safer and more effective?

If a woman is classified as estrogen deficient, which is a rare state, then the need for estrogen is clinically indicated in a bio-identical form, not in a synthetic form. The proper use of bio-identical hormones is safe and should be encouraged.

WOMEN AND HEART ATTACKS

Women experience heart attacks very differently than men, making it more difficult to diagnose and treat them. Women can have a heart attack and not even know it. About 35 percent of all heart attacks in women go unnoticed and unreported. A woman's heart will go into sudden vasospasm. This occurs due to a drop in estrogen and progesterone as we move into menopause. This is why young women, sometimes in their forties, will just drop dead having never had a symptom. Menopause is occurring earlier today than in the past, a fact that may explain why such heart problems are affecting younger women.

Men's heart attacks, on the other hand, are due to insulin and cortisol dysfunction. Their arteries become clogged (coronary artery occlusion). As men's bodies are aging and developing heart disease, their kidneys are being affected by constant water retention from high carbohydrate diets. This water retention often leads to hypertension as well. Only 50 percent of coronary artery disease deaths are associated with major blocked arteries. Therefore, the other 50 percent must be from something else.

Excessive sugar intake is now recognized as the number one risk factor for heart attacks in women, and number two for men. Excessive animal fat intake is number two for women and number one for men. This is due, in part, to the fact that just one teaspoon of sugar impairs the immune system by about 40 percent. Many Americans are consuming an average of two or more teaspoons of sugar every hour all day long, which keeps their immunity constantly low.

THE HORMONE CONNECTION

Levels of hormones change as women age, which is why the goal to keep hormones balanced is crucial in preventing breast cancer, heart disease and other maladies. Premenopausal women who suffer from vasospasm lack progesterone. This type of heart attack damages the heart by constricting and shutting off blood flow. When the heart muscle lacks blood and oxygen, it dies.

Researchers at the Oregon Regional Primate Research Center of Reproductive Sciences removed the ovaries of rhesus monkeys whose hearts were young and healthy. They made up cocktails of vasospasm-inducing substances from the blood of women who had experienced vasospasm, which was a formula for death. Five out of the seven monkeys died. When they used HRT under the same circumstances, they reported that estrogen plus progestins did not protect them from coronary vasospasm, but natural estrogen (17-beta estradiol) plus natural progesterone did.

his is another example supporting the evidence that natural hormones work without serious side effects. Therefore, the science that supports conventional hormone replacement therapy as a means to protect against osteoporosis, heart disease, stroke and menopausal symptoms (such as hot flashes, depression, sleep disturbances and vaginal dryness) can be tossed in the trash.

In view of the acknowledgement of the dangers of synthetic hormones versus the protection gained from natural hormones, women can now be relieved to know that these drugs are *not* safe, nor do they replicate the body's own production of hormones. We also know that the synthetic route of replacing hormones causes an *increase* in stroke and heart attacks.

THE CHOLESTEROL FARCE

Christie Ballantyne, M.D., a cardiologist with the Baylor College of Medicine, said that most of her heart disease patients have a total cholesterol level of less than 240. And she added: *"The majority of people who end up having heart attacks or strokes don't have high cholesterol."*

This flies in the face of the National Cholesterol Education Program (NCEP) chieftans who have one goal in mind and that is to lower the cholesterol levels of Americans, whether it's beneficial or not. This is also one way to turn healthy people into patients.

Contrary to popular belief, high cholesterol levels do *not* cause heart disease. It is an unproven theory.

With that said, institutions across this country are spending billions of tax dollars in support of this claim.

According to the American Journal of the College of Nutrition, *"Many studies reported over the past two years have shown that dietary cholesterol is not a significant factor in an individual's plasma cholesterol level or in cardiovascular disease risk. Reports from the Lipid Research Clinics Research Prevalence Study and the Framingham Heart Study have shown that dietary cholesterol is not related to either blood cholesterol levels or heart disease deaths."*

Dr. Michael E. DeBakey, famous heart surgeon and Chancellor Emeritus at Baylor College of Medicine, Houston, Texas, conducted a study of 1,700 patients who had atherosclerosis severe enough for hospitalization. Only one out of five patients had high cholesterol. That means 80 percent of the patients did not have high cholesterol, but had heart disease anyway.

The National Heart, Lung and Blood Institute's Honolulu Heart Program began an on-going study in 1965 involving more than 8,000 men. Dr. Kendrick states this quote as it appeared in the *Lancet* medical journal: *"Our data accord with previous findings of increased mortality in elderly people with low serum cholesterol, and show that long-term persistence of low cholesterol concentration actually increases the risk of death."*

Whoa! Low cholesterol concentration can actually increase the risk of death?

The new NCEP guidelines for cholesterol levels call for a target LDL of 70 for heart patients who are considered to be at very high risk of a heart attack. High risk or not, 70 is an extremely low LDL level; it will be almost impossible for anyone to hit that level without using statin drugs, which the NCEP recommends as a course of action. The *Lancet* lends us a grand opportunity to take advantage of a long term study that we often do not have access to, yet the NCEP has totally ignored this rich data.

Consider this analogy. Would you purchase a new home if you only had access to what the front of the house looked like without the benefit of looking inside to see what else the home had to offer? Of course not. Then why would we consider the recommendations of the NCEP, looking at LDL only as the culprit to heart disease and making national recommendations based on statements about LDL, when there are multiple factors that are markers for heart disease? This is the HRT story all over again.

Cholesterol is a fat-soluble steroid from which all of the steroid hormones are made; steroid hormones include cortisol, cortisone, aldosterone in the adrenal glands, progesterone, estrogen and testosterone. One role of these hormones is to protect nerves and nerve impulse propagation for enhancement of brain function. So if cholesterol is too low, the brain will suffer. Cholesterol is a risk marker for cardiovascular disease, not the cause.

Cholesterol is excreted from the liver in the form of a secretion known as bile; it sometimes crystallizes in the gall bladder to form gallstones. Cholesterol is also the precursor to vitamin D, and is necessary for numerous biochemical processes including mineral metabolism. The bile salts, required for the digestion of fat, are made of cholesterol. If cholesterol levels are too low, digesting fats could become a problem. Cholesterol also functions as a powerful antioxidant, thus protecting us against cancer and aging.

The liver manufactures about 2 grams of cholesterol per day; most of this cholesterol is made from sugars and refined starches and is used for an assortment of biochemical processes. A small amount is absorbed from food in the small intestines, but this quantity is needed by the body to give it the substrates necessary to manufacture enough cholesterol. Eliminating cholesterol foods from one's diet is therefore ill advised.

Smaller amounts of cholesterol are manufactured by our intestines and body cells. If this substance is so terribly dangerous, then why does the body produce the majority of it? It's because the body cannot function without proper levels of cholesterol. We obviously need cholesterol to function; to chemically alter the production of this valuable substance is dangerous.

Here are several reasons why we need cholesterol:
- cholesterol is used to help construct protective cell membranes,
- it provides the basis of the steroid hormones produced in the adrenal glands, ovaries and testes,
- it helps your body make vitamin D, which we are learning is more beneficial for other conditions and diseases than we had determined in the past,
- it is necessary for brain function,
- it is required for efficiency to store sugar and starch calories,
- it helps cells maintain their shape and acts as a barrier to protect certain liquids and water from leaving your body too quickly, and
- it supports the myelin sheath that protects nerves.

HIGH-DENSITY LIPOPROTEINS (HDL) VERSUS LOW-DENSITY LIPOPROTEINS (LDL) CHOLESTEROL

HDL cholesterol has been found to protect against heart disease whereas LDL has been found to be predictive of heart disease. These proteins carry cholesterol in serum. HDL helps to move cholesterol through the arterial walls protecting it from attaching. LDL, on the other hand, is not so beneficial. When and if it becomes oxidized (combined with oxygen), it can damage the arterial walls, thus setting the stage for mineral and fat deposits. Keeping LDL levels lower may be one of the most important things you can do to protect against heart disease.

Lowering LDL levels can be done safely through lifestyle changes, exercise, diet and nutritional supplementation, *not* through drugs.

WHY THE CHOLESTEROL-HEART DISEASE THEORY IS WRONG

Ancel Keys, Ph.D., Professor Emeritus of Public Health at the University of Minnesota, was a pioneer in the development of a field that combines physiology, nutrition, epidemiology and prevention.

If you haven't noticed by now, I have an affinity toward pioneers and their work. Rarely are they influenced by financial or political motivation, but rather by a passion to seek the truth. Much of Keys' work was done in the area of cardiology and epidemiology.

Dr. Keys turned 100 on January 26, 2004, and passed away in November 2004. He was a health and nutrition researcher who espoused and adopted a Mediterranean diet years ago. It evidently served him well.

*T*his is what Keys said about the connection between cholesterol in the diet and cholesterol in the blood. *"There's no connection whatsoever between cholesterol in food and cholesterol in blood. And we've known that all along. Cholesterol in the diet doesn't matter at all unless you happen to be a chicken or a rabbit."*

Prior to Keys' death, Mark Becker, Assistant Vice President and Dean of the University School of Public Health had this to say about Keys: *"He is simply a public health giant." Few figures in the 20th century, if any, can match his contributions to the biology and epidemiology of coronary heart disease."*

Dr. George Mann, Ph.D., M.D., is a retired Professor of Medicine from Vanderbilt University. He was trained as a nutritional biochemist and as a physician. He states categorically: *"The diet-heart hypothesis has been repeatedly shown to be wrong, and yet, for complicated reasons of pride, profit, and prejudice, the hypothesis continues to be exploited by scientists, fund-raising enterprises, food companies, and even governmental agencies. The public is being deceived by the greatest health scam of the century."*

So why does conventional medicine insist that dietary cholesterol is the culprit? The quote above is quite telling. You will be well-served to follow the research and writings of these brilliant scientists and learn the real truth behind the value of nutrition and how it directly affects your health.

PITFALLS OF CONVENTIONAL ASSUMPTIONS

By now, you should be getting about as frustrated as I am, having seen the neatly knitted pattern medical institutions in this country are weaving regarding women's health. Actually this pattern is affecting all consumers. Neurotic behavior is one way to explain their thinking.

Neurotics engage in extreme behavior in defense of the behavior itself. Even though we experience positive results repeatedly from natural approaches to health and healing, the current mindset refuses to accept this as "good medicine." It does not fit neatly into conventional medicine's comfort zone of the double-blind method of testing.

Remember, however, the way our institutions are set up today. Only with double-blind studies can a therapy or drug be patentable, thus placing total control into the hands of the pharmaceutical industry, one of the largest monopolies in existence today. The FDA, whose responsibility is to protect the consumer from dangerous foods and drugs, appears to be little more than the enforcement arm of the major drug companies.

Approximately 85 percent of all therapies and procedures that are commonly used by physicians and in hospitals have *never* received any kind of rigorous evaluation. Only 17 to 20 percent of conventional medical practices are based on scientifically validated evidence. Eighty percent are based on anecdotal data. Is this a double standard?

Dr. David A. Grimes, M.D., of the University of California, San Francisco School of Medicine, states, *"[M]uch if not most of contemporary medical practice still lacks a scientific foundation".* He provides examples such as radial keratotomy, laparoscopic vaginal hysterectomy and episiotomy.

Dr. Marcia Angell, M.D., the former interim editor-in-chief of the *New England Journal of Medicine* (NEJM) resigned from her position in June 2000. She decided to walk away from this prestigious position to write a book about the stronghold that drug companies have over clinical trials and the way medicine is practiced today. She has this to say:

"The most startling fact in 2002 is that the combined profits for the ten drug companies in the Fortune 500 ($35.9 billion) were more than the profits for all the other 490 businesses put together ($33.7 billion). When I say this is a profitable industry, I mean really profitable. It is difficult to conceive of how awash in money big pharma is."

The healing model of medicine observes with great discernment the outcomes of the double-blind method of testing, in conjunction with clinical experience, observation, (empirical), anecdotal/self reporting data and actual facts. Natural approaches are ultimately safer and more effective.

Surgery...Is it really good medicine?

By now you have observed and learned, with great consternation, that medicine is driven by economics and politics. It certainly does not stop with surgery. Some heart specialists across the country are struggling. There are conflicting views within the medical establishment regarding treatments for heart disease. Naturally, the different sides argue that their approach is best. This is not a very good scenario for consumers, who are at their mercy.

We know through a large body of scientific evidence that heart disease is preventable and can, in most cases, be managed and reversed through lifestyle choices. Unfortunately, this is *not* the model of prevention that is making the headlines.

Follow the dollar. Dr. Thomas B. Graboys, Associate Clinical Professor of Medicine at Brigham and Women's Hospital and Harvard Medical School (Boston), says it succinctly, *"The bottom line is economics. The high reimbursements for angioplasty and bypass surgeries all contribute to the cash cow. All over the country, hospitals are going under. This is the currency that keeps them salvageable."*

This candid comment is disconcerting. And don't think this does not apply to other surgical procedures women have endured over the years.

Of course, hospitals are going under. There are entirely too many hospitals in some communities that are operating at 20 to 30 percent capacity. Regardless of this scenario, the medical community is more concerned about displacing medical personnel than making some hard core business decisions that would benefit the entire community.

Since heart surgery is such a popular procedure these days (and we know why) the issue of safety is often overlooked. Any type of surgery poses risks. Throughout this book, the idea I have been trying to get across is: consider the benefit to risk ratio before making any healthcare decision.

Catheterization carries a risk of heart attack, stroke or death in about 1 in 600. Other risks include kidney damage, allergic reaction to the dye, irregular heartbeat, infection and damage to the blood vessels. For women, particularly those over the age of 75 or those who have diabetes, this procedure carries an even greater risk.

It's one thing when there is a life or death situation; however, the majority of decisions in healthcare are based upon a community standard. This "standard" means that whatever peers are doing is the accepted practice, whether or not it is the best.

As an example, 1 in 3 arteries close again within weeks after an angioplasty procedure whereby a stent is used to hold open the ballooned artery. Even the American Heart Association and the American College of Cardiology agree that these invasive procedures should not be considered a first line of defense. With the number of heart procedures done in this country, this can only be interpreted as paying lip service.

The frustration for those of us who endorse and promote the model of a gentler, safer, more natural medicine lies in the fact that even the physicians who agree that surgery should not be the first line of defense make the decision to use medications as an alternative. Medications, of course, are not necessarily the answer either. Many other options, such as lifestyle behavior changes, are far superior in safety, costs and long term outcomes.

Physicians are not the only guilty party. Consumers want quick fixes and immediate symptom relief. Many are not willing to revamp their lifestyles and are enamored by the concept of high tech medicine. Insurance coverage and malpractice suits further complicate the situation. And when someone else is footing the bill, the sky is the limit.

Women need to re-evaluate all recommendations made by

their personal physicians, especially when drugs and/or surgery are being discussed as a means of intervention. If this crystal clear example does not open eyes, chances are, nothing will.

And Then Came the Statins

Groundbreaking news came from one of our prestigious journals that statin drugs in high doses are the answer to lowering cholesterol to protect consumers from the risk of heart disease. Oddly, what was *not* mentioned were the serious side affects that can result from the use of statins. Based on previous studies about cholesterol, why does medicine focus on cholesterol as the single culprit?

Many studies have reported a direct link to neuropathy, dizziness, heart failure, cognitive impairment, cancer, pancreatitis and depression from the use of statin drugs. Commentators across the globe have reported that only 11 million Americans are currently taking statins, when actually 36 million should be. This misinformation could have far reaching effects. These drugs have not been around long enough to observe the real long term effects, yet they are being recommended for a lifetime.

"Carcinogenicity of Lipid-Lowering Drugs" was the title of an article reporting that the two most popular classes of lipid-lowering drugs cause cancer in rodents. The jury is still out on humans and the cancer connection. However, based upon the deception and manipulation of data that occurs in scientific trials of all colors, it would be best to avoid these drugs until more definitive, longitudinal studies have been completed.

Statin drugs not only inhibit the production of cholesterol, but they also inhibit a whole family of intermediary substances. Many of these substances have important biochemical functions in their own right. Statins block the action of an enzyme that produces cholesterol. They also cause the body to excrete more cholesterol through the intestine or stool.

It is true that statins lower cholesterol levels, but what does this have to do with being healthy? We just learned earlier about the vital role cholesterol plays in our bodies. Don't kid yourself; these drugs are more harmful than you have been led to believe. Up until now, no one has been able to show that lowering cholesterol levels through the use of statin drugs improves the quality of life or extends life span. These drugs cause liver damage, muscle problems and cardiac damage. Statin drugs affect the brain also. We are not able to make enough estrogen and progesterone, as needed for neurotransmitters in the brain, when taking statins.

If your doctor prescribes the following medications, *BEWARE:* Lipitor (atorvastatin), Zocor (simvastatin), Mevacor (lovastatin), and Pravachol (pravastatin). Also note that another statin, Baycol (cerivastatin), was withdrawn from the market in August 2001, due to 31 deaths from a muscle-wasting disease. Baycol, like other statins, did not offer much benefit. It gained popularity because of aggressive pricing and marketing, not because of its safety, efficacy or health benefits.

Please remember, cholesterol does not cause heart disease. Studies prove this beyond a doubt. If your cholesterol is already in the "normal" or "low" range, it means you're a prime candidate/target to be drugged. Beware, ladies. No study has shown a significant reduction in mortality in women treated with statins.

The University of British Columbia Therapeutics Initiative came to the same conclusion, with the finding that statins offer no benefit to women for prevention of heart disease.

Yet, many women on Premarin are being prescribed these drugs. The side effects of these statin drugs are dangerous in the long run. We have no idea about the long term effects on women when statins are combined with Premarin.

The statin drugs correct plasma lipid levels optimally, yet the real magnitude of their benefits is marginal and certainly not better than attained with agents that do not effect plasma lipid levels. Some of the recommendations and actions relating to plasma cholesterol levels, and to atherosclerosis, are based on concepts that are fundamentally flawed and need to be revised.

In February 2004, *Circulation* published an article in which more than twenty organizations endorsed cardiovascular disease prevention guidelines for women with several mentions of "preferably a statin." Well, perhaps this recommendation should be rescinded.

Groundbreaking news hit the headlines this past year about Zocor, Merck's best selling cholesterol-lowering drug, that reported sales of $2.7 billion worldwide in the first six months of 2004. No conclusive benefits were experienced with Zocor over the benefits of a low-cholesterol diet combined with a low dose of Zocor in preventing heart attacks and deaths. The study was supported by a grant from Merck & Company. Is the fox guarding the hen house?

Some medical authorities are commending the researchers for publishing the study's findings even though the results were less than favorable. Isn't this their job? Their thinking is that they have been vindicated this time by telling the truth rather than sweeping the information under the rug. So what about all the other studies where less than favorable results have not been reported? Studies are conducted to help us determine whether or not an intervention has a greater benefit than risk.

The average consumer may not think much about these recommendations or guidelines, or may be too naïve or complacent to care; however, they should definitely beware. Studies have shown that low cholesterol levels are directly linked to depression, aggression, violent behavior, suicide, increased risk of stroke and poor immune function.

The next time you read or hear any news about the value of statins and their ability to lower cholesterol and protect you from heart disease, read between the lines and run. This push on statin usage only benefits those who are marketing and selling the drugs. You now have the science that backs up the truth, so do not be fooled.

A HEARTY PRO-ACTIVE APPROACH

The evidence is overwhelming. Using a drug or any foreign substance to manipulate the production of hormones, cholesterol or any substance the body produces is risky business. Lowering cholesterol levels has nothing to do with heart disease. Therefore, a wholistic approach of lifestyle changes involving exercise, diet and nutritional supplementation and relaxation are the key.

Other indicators leading to the increase of heart disease are:

- Nutritional deficiencies
- Hormone imbalance
- Stress
- Lack of exercise
- Obesity
- Genetics

A GOOD NUTRITIONAL FOUNDATION

Unhealthy food selections are the crux of modern day diseases. The foods that contribute to heart disease are called atherogenic. Fats, sugars and starches, when consumed in excessive amounts, are the foods that create the manifestation of health conditions that eventually turn into chronic diseases.

We'll start with saturated fats since they are a major

contributing factor to heart disease. The fats I'm talking about, however, are the ones that are foreign and toxic to our bodies. Over time, excessive consumption causes the body to degenerate at the cellular level.

Hydrogenation of oils known as trans fats have wreaked havoc in our bodies. Since these fats are contained in the majority of processed foods (please read labels), heart disease rates have increased more than 50 percent over the past several years. I discussed this briefly in previous chapters.

In fact, the consumption of these oils and fats in the past few decades has been marketed as a way to *decrease* risks of heart disease. This has been disastrous for the consumer.

The low-fat and non-fat diets that are full of artificial ingredients are alluring because they have been marketed as quick fixes. This is how twisted the marketing of health information has become.

*H*ydrogenated coconut, cottonseed and palm kernel oils are the most common plant oils marketed as cholesterol-free. Don't be fooled. What you are not being told is that through the process of hydrogenation, these oils end up as saturated fats that are unfamiliar to our body's metabolism. Hydrogenation is a process whereby an extra hydrogen atom is pressed with high pressure. This process creates a different type of fat molecule that is not found in the human food chain. These fats deplete the body of essential fatty acids and are linked to cardiovascular disease and cancer. So when you see a food marketed as fat-free, cholesterol-free, hydrogenated or partially hydrogenated, *don't* buy it. It's junk food.

These oils, along with other fats from feed-lot animals and cows milk, do not metabolize very well and end up as LDL cholesterol, which is more likely to clog our arteries. Studies beginning in the 1950s began showing these hardened, processed oils as dangerous. Margarine is in the same category. Switch to butter and use it in moderation. Our bodies know how to metabolize this fat. It is not foreign.

As of late, there are several butter substitutes from vegetable and other sources that are being touted as healthy. They may be, but my suggestion is to stay away from any substitutes unless you have an allergic reaction or sensitivity to the "real food" or there is ample scientific evidence that supports safety and overall benefits of the substitute.

When substitutes are introduced into the diet, people have a tendency to consume more than they should. This has happened with diet foods, diet sodas, low-fat and non-fat foods.

Some of the more popular brands of butter substitutes include: I Can't Believe It's Not Butter, Smart Balance and Earth Balance Soy Garden. They are recommended to help lower cholesterol levels or are marketed as low-fat. As you have learned, however, the "real thing" is what the body thrives on.

If you are consuming these products because you like the taste, that's another story. Don't count on them to necessarily help you avoid illness, disease and other conditions. And be sure to read the labels very closely. What appears to be natural or safe, may not be so at all. Don't forget that lowering cholesterol is not the answer to the chronic illnesses and conditions we have addressed.

ARE ALL FATS BAD?

There is great confusion about the types of fats that should be consumed and what types are considered heart healthy. To simplify this entire topic I will make a few suggestions and provide some guidelines that will help you decide what is best for you and your family.

OLIVE OIL

You can't go wrong with virgin olive oil. It is the first press from the olive, is minimally processed, and possesses a high degree of protection against oxidation. The Greeks, Italians and all cultures in the Mediterranean have used this oil for centuries.

Researchers have observed with great consternation that Greeks who consume large amounts of olive oil have an extremely low incidence of hardening of the arteries. Further research has shown that olive oil is digested like complex carbohydrates and has healthful fatty acids that contribute to heart health.

GRAPESEED OIL.

We don't hear too much about this oil, but it has been used in Europe for years and is considered a favorite. This oil has a light, delicate taste, which enhances other flavors rather than dominating them. It is a byproduct of wine production. This oil's extremely high smoke point permits high-heat cooking, including smokeless frying and sautéing, without destroying the integrity of the oil.

Some studies have demonstrated that grapeseed oil may also be effective in correcting blood cholesterol levels in certain individuals, thereby reducing their risk of cardiac events. It is also known to have improved serum cholesterol levels.

We need to focus not only on total cholesterol levels, but also on LDL, HDL and total cholesterol ratio. Grapeseed oil appears to reduce LDL so it can be carried to the liver for elimination. It is also known to be a natural source of vitamin E and essential fatty acids necessary for normal cell metabolism.

NATURAL COCONUT OIL.

I don't mean hydrogenated coconut oil, so please don't get confused. Coconut oil is one of the healthiest oils you can consume. It is rich in lauric acid, which is known for being antiviral, antibacterial and antifungal, contains no trans fats and boosts the immune system.

Jon J. Kabara, Ph.D, Professor Emeritus, Michigan State University, states that the medium chain fats found in coconut oil (lauric acid) are similar to fats in mothers' milk and have similar nutriceutical effects, such as protecting infants from infections. You can even use it on your skin to help prevent wrinkles. Unlike other oils, coconut oil that has been kept at room temperature for a year has been tested for rancidity and showed no evidence of it.

Consumers who use coconut oil have experienced remarkable physiological effects (as antihistamines, anti-infectives, antiseptics, promoters of immunity, glucocorticoid antagonist, nontoxic anticancer agents, for example), which may not be surprising because of the high lauric acid content.

As far as the evidence goes, coconut oil, added regularly to a balanced diet, lowers cholesterol to normal by promoting its conversion into pregnenolone. Coconut-eating cultures in the tropics have consistently lower cholesterol than people in the U.S. The cultures that use coconut oil regularly have cholesterol levels of about 160, while eating mainly cholesterol rich foods (eggs, milk, cheese, meat, shellfish). It has also been reported that coconut oil can actually help lower cholesterol, improve diabetic conditions, reduce weight and reduce the risk of heart disease.

A study published in 1981 reported that the populations of two South Pacific islands were examined over a period of time starting in the 1960s, before Western foods were prevalent in the diets of either culture. The study was designed to investigate the relative effects of saturated fat and dietary cholesterol in determining serum cholesterol levels. Coconuts were practically a staple in the island diets, with up to 60 percent of their caloric intake coming from the saturated fat of coconut oil. The study found very lean and healthy people who were relatively free from the modern diseases of Western cultures, including obesity. Their conclusion: *"Vascular disease is uncommon in both populations and there is no evidence of the high saturated fat intake having a harmful effect in these populations."*

Try introducing coconut oil into your diet to enjoy the benefits. The cholesterol-lowering properties of coconut oil are a direct result of its ability to stimulate thyroid function. In the presence of adequate thyroid hormone, cholesterol (specifically LDL-cholesterol) is converted by enzymatic processes to the vitally necessary anti-aging steroids, pregnenolone, progesterone and DHEA. These substances are required to help prevent heart disease, senility, obesity, cancer and other diseases associated with aging and chronic degenerative diseases.

LET'S NOT FORGET THE OMEGA-3'S

I discussed omega-3's in previous chapters. However, it's important to learn about their benefits as they are directly related to heart disease.

Omega-3 fatty acids have been shown in several studies to be protective of heart disease and particularly cardiac arrest.

The Greenland Eskimos consume diets very high in fat from seals, whales, and fish, yet have a low rate of coronary heart disease. The fats the Eskimos consume contain large quantities of the very-long-chain and highly polyunsaturated fatty acids of EPA and DHA, which are abundant in fish, shellfish, and sea mammals, yet are scarce or absent in land animals and plants. EPA and DHA are synthesized by phytoplankton. These are the plants of the waters and are the base of the food chain for marine life.

The point being, omega-3 fatty acids are an essential part of a woman's diet. Oftentimes, women experience a variety of skin problems such as eczema, cracked heels and thick patches of skin. This can be directly related to a deficiency of omega-3 fatty acids. Green leafy vegetables, flaxseeds, pumpkin seeds and nuts, and wild game are rich in omega-3's.

A deficiency in omega-3's can also impair cell membrane function, and since the brain is the richest source of fatty acids, which influence neurotransmitter synthesis, it is critical that people consume rich sources of them. Although I am not a big fan of consuming fish oil as a supplement over foods, it's becoming a more suitable means these days of getting the omega-3's, due to the risk of mercury in the fresh fish today. If you have access to wild Alaskan salmon, this is a tasty means of consuming good healthy oils.

Adding omega-3's to your daily diet will substantially lower your risk of heart disease by lowering LDL cholesterol and triglycerides. They can also help prevent and reduce the risk of certain cancers, including breast cancer.

As always, never overdo a good thing. Strive for a balance when consuming food. The more natural the food, the greater the benefits.

THE SKINNY ON SUGARS

I must report once again, that contrary to what you hear in the news and from some of the most prestigious medical institutions and journals in this country about fat causing heart disease, that is not the total, true picture. What poses a far greater risk is the excessive consumption of sugars and starches from simple carbohydrates.

*O*ur culture consumes entirely too many sweets, potatoes, white rice, white breads and snack foods that are highly processed. As a result of our insatiable appetite for sweets, a rapid rise in blood glucose levels occurs. Constant insulin is then required to lower the rise in blood sugar. The production of too much insulin makes it difficult for the body to lose fat and excess weight, which has been classified as a contributing factor to heart disease.

Pure whole sugar cane actually contains some healthful ingredients such as magnesium, vitamin B6, chromium, other B vitamins and fiber. A major problem with the kind of sugar found in candy, fruit drinks, soda pops, etc. is that it's heavily processed and stripped of its nutritive value. There is nothing natural about it. So unless you eat whole powdered sugar cane, sugar will not be very good for you.

Too much sugar can lead to tooth decay, obesity, and adult-onset diabetes. As mentioned earlier in this chapter, too much sugar can also impair your immune system, making it harder to fight off illness and infection.

Fructose, which is found naturally in fruit, is often promoted as being healthier and safer than refined sugars. However, there is more to this story. Takasago Municipal Hospital in Japan reported that fructose is associated with the progression of diabetic complications.

Fructose, however, has a very low glycemic index, meaning that it has very little effect on blood sugars when used in small amounts. The key is to avoid excessive use of this sweetener.

Fructose has no enzymes, vitamins, or minerals. It robs the body of its micronutrient treasures in order to assimilate itself for physiological use. Fructose reduces the affinity of insulin for its receptor. This is the first step for glucose to enter a cell and be metabolized. As a result, the body needs to pump out more insulin to handle the same amount of glucose.

Linus Pauling, Ph.D., noted winner of two Nobel Prizes, the 1954 award for Chemistry and the 1962 Nobel Peace Prize, reported many years ago that refined carbohydrates, not fat, are the culprit in obesity. These carbohydrates quickly break down into sugars and cause a rise in glucose levels, almost as high as simple sugars. As these simple carbohydrates and sugars are consumed on a regular basis, the pancreas continues to produce insulin. When too much insulin is produced, LDL cholesterol levels and triglycerides increase.

Over time, insulin is no longer able to do its job of getting the glucose into the cells; therefore, insulin resistance occurs. Insulin resistance and Type 2 diabetes are some of the major causes of obesity that, in turn, contribute to an increased risk of heart disease. Perhaps you can now understand why the incidence of Type 2 diabetes is increasing in this country.

Now you can see the direct relationship of sugars and simple carbohydrates and how they contribute to obesity and heart disease. What's important to keep in mind is that sugar and simple carbohydrates are not as benign as most people think. This is not a reason, however, to eliminate *all* carbohydrates. The carbo-free frenzy is not the answer either.

It should be no surprise, once you understand how sugar is metabolized, why America is struggling with the epidemic of obesity. Consume sugars and starches in moderation and do your best to read labels. Know what you are consuming. Artificial sugars are an absolute *no* because of their link to many chronic illnesses and diseases.

Xylitol... Every sweet tooth's dream

Xylitol is a natural substance and natural sweetener found in fibrous vegetables and fruits and comes from the birch tree. It is a crystalline carbohydrate that is classified in some chemical encyclopedia as a sugar. It is a naturally occurring form of the 5-carbon sugar, xylose, which is quite different from sorbitol, which is a 6-carbon hexitol. Sorbitol supports the cavity-causing bacteria in the mouth, whereas xylitol actually prevents cavities.

Xylitol was discovered in 1891 by a German chemist, Emil Fisher. It was not until the sugar shortages became a reality that Finland began to use xylitol. Those who began using it were also known to have better health stimulated the desire to research the reason why.

There are several benefits to using xylitol. Those who consume xylitol on a regular basis have fewer cavities, improved periodontal health (gum health), and a reduction in sinus and throat infections, bad breath, gastric and duondenal ulcers and H. pylori. This is a dentist's dream.

Many researchers believe that xylitol mints, gum or nasal spray may be a safe and easy way to treat and prevent chronic sinusitis and more serious throat and lung infections. Some studies have shown it to reduce the incidence of middle ear infections in children by 40 percent.

Because xylitol is slowly metabolized, it is a natural insulin stabilizer, which does not cause an abrupt rise and fall of blood sugar like sugar does. Foods sweetened with xylitol will not raise insulin levels, thus making it a perfect sweetener for diabetics and those who want to lose weight.

To be fully effective, xylitol should be used daily. Much of the research suggests consuming at least 4 to12 grams per day which equates to about 4 to12 mints or pieces of gum per day. It should be used after each meal and after the mouth has been rinsed with cold water. Other researchers suggest consuming more, depending on what type of pending condition may exist or what it is a consumer wants to accomplish from a preventive perspective.

Xylitol gets my vote. I have used it in recipes that my friends give rave reviews. Xylitol is approved as a food additive in the U.S., not as a sweetener. It is a safe and healthy choice for those who are watching their weight.

STEVIA, THE SWEET SAFE SUBSTITUTE

Stevia, is a perennial shrub native to the Amambay mountain region in Paraguay and has actually been shown to lower blood pressure and improve insulin sensitivity. The Japanese and Brazilians have been consuming it for over 20 years; it has been approved as a safe, natural and non-caloric sweetener in those countries. The Japanese use stevia to sweeten everything from soy sauce to pickles, confections, and soft drinks. They are also the largest consumer of stevia leaves and extracts in the world.

Even multinational giants like Coca-Cola and Beatrice Foods use stevia extracts (as a replacement for NutraSweet and saccharin) to sweeten foods they sell in Japan, Brazil, and other countries where it is approved as a food additive. Not so in the United States, however, where stevia is specifically prohibited from use as a sweetener or as a food additive. Why? Many people believe that the national non-caloric sweetener giants have been successful in preventing this all-natural, inexpensive, and non-patentable sweetener from being used to replace their patented, synthetic, more expensive sweeteners.

Stevia can be found in local health food stores and is a very popular product for those who are informed. Using the Internet, go to Google.com and type in "Stevia." You will find several interesting and informative pieces of literature related to this sweetener.

Since the mid-1980s, the FDA has labeled stevia an "unsafe food additive" and gone to extensive lengths to keep it off the U.S. market — including initiating a search-and-seizure campaign and full-fledged "import alert." So adamant has the FDA remained on the subject, that even though stevia can now be legally marketed as a dietary supplement under legislation enacted in 1994, any mention of its possible use as a sweetener is still strictly prohibited.

Instead of protecting the public health and environment, we routinely see the FDA give in to business, no matter who or what gets hurt.

Rob McCaleb, president and founder of the Herb Research Foundation, comments: *"Sweetness is big money. Nobody wants to see something cheap and easy to grow on the market competing with the things they worked so hard to get approved."* It's the same story over and over again; economics and politics over health and safety.

SPLENDA IS *NOT* SO SPENDID

Splenda has been marketed in this country as the latest and greatest brand name substitute sweetener for sugar-derivative sucralose. Sucralose is produced by chlorinating sugar (sucrose). This involves chemically changing the structure of the sugar molecules by substituting three chlorine atoms for three hydroxyl groups. Molecularly, it is converted from cane sugar to a non-calorie sweetener and is not recognized as sugar by the body.

We have learned from previous chapters how changing the molecular structure of a natural product wreaks havoc on the body.

Splenda is marketed as low-carb and no-calorie without full disclosure of the whole story, yet the headlines make it sound quite alluring. There have been no long term studies conducted on this man-made product, yet it has been approved by the

FDA. Another double standard makes its mark again.

According to a MEDLINE search, the following number of studies have been conducted on artificial sweeteners:

SUBSTITUTE	# OF STUDIES
Saccharin	2,374
Aspartame	598
Cyclamates	459
Acesulfame-K	28
Sucralose	19

The International Food Information Council has the following to say about sucralose: *"Sucralose is produced by chlorinating sugar (sucrose). This involves chemically changing the structure of the sugar molecules by substituting three chlorine atoms for three hydroxyl groups."*

Science confirms that when a chemical is structurally changed, the body does not know how to metabolize it. So why are consumers being fooled into thinking this is such a safe product?

It's the marketing and special interest groups pursuing their own interests that inevitably lead to decisions that are not in the best interest of the consumer. It's also interesting that the International Food Information Council states: *Sucralose has an excellent safety profile. More than 100 scientific studies conducted over a 20-year period (contrary to the MEDLINE search) demonstrate that sucralose is safe for use as a sweetening ingredient. The data from the studies were independently evaluated by international experts in a variety of scientific disciplines, including toxicology, oncology, teratology, neurology, hematology, pediatrics and nutrition. Importantly, comprehensive toxicology studies, designed to meet the highest scientific standards, have clearly demonstrated that sucralose is not carcinogenic.*

According to *Consumers' Research Magazine,* sucralose provides some benefits for the corporations making and using it, but not for consumers. They state, *"But are such foods truly beneficial and desirable? Diabetics, weight watchers, and the general public might make better food choices by selecting basic, rather than highly processed foods; for example, apples, rather than turnovers; or plain, rather than sweetened, dairy foods."*

They note that non-caloric artificial sweeteners are not replacing, but are supplementing, conventional sweeteners. They note that as of 1990, Americans were consuming an average of 20 pounds (sugar sweetness equivalency) of artificial sweeteners, and as consumption of sugar-substitutes has risen, so too has consumption of sugar.

So there you have it, ladies. Like I mentioned earlier, substitutes are rarely consumed in moderation and often accompany the "real food" in addition. You have heard it from the scientists. Stay away from any sugars or foods that have been molecularly altered. Regardless of what the FDA says, do not believe that the use of artificial chemicals is safe. Exercise caution because there will be a price to pay in the long run, and it will not be cheap. There is a good chance your health will be at risk once again.

SUPPLEMENTS FOR HEART DISEASE

If you were told that you could fight heart disease, viruses and other chronic illnesses and diseases by using a simple supplement, would you buy it? If I share with you the research that supports this concept, will you still buy it, even though medical institutions and the government tell you it is dangerous and worthless? Let's explore further.

The use of supplements for preventing and healing heart disease has been known for several years. The theory that heart disease is related to a deficiency of vitamin C was first proposed by G.C. Willis, M.D. in 1953. He discovered that atherosclerotic plaques form over vitamin C-starved tissues in guinea pigs and humans.

In 1989, Linus Pauling, Ph.D., and his associate Matthias Rath, M.D., formulated a unified theory of heart disease and discovered the cure. They discovered that only one form of cholesterol, *Lp(a)*, (an LDL-like cholesterol substance) creates plaques over the arterial lesions. *Lp(a)* also has lysine and proline receptors. The *Lp(a)* binding inhibitors became the Pauling Therapy (increase the concentration of these essential and non-toxic amino acids in the blood serum) to treat heart disease. Vitamin C, lysine and proline in high dosages become binding inhibitors that restore vascular health and destroy arterial plaque. *"Vitamin C is essential for the building of collagen, the most abundant protein and the major component of connective tissue. This connective tissue has structural and supportive functions which are indispensable to heart tissue, to blood vessels- in fact, to all tissues. Collagen is not only the most abundant protein in our bodies, it also occurs in larger amounts than all other proteins put together. It cannot be built without vitamin C. No heart, or blood vessel or other organ can possibly perform its functions without collagen. No heart or blood vessel can be maintained in healthy condition without vitamin C."* — Roger J. Williams, Ph.D., a world-renowned biochemist specializing in nutrition, Biochemical Individuality, and Public Education.

Cellular Medicine, a term used by Dr. Matthias Rath, is the solution to heart disease. The main role of heart muscle cells is to pump and maintain blood circulation. The smooth muscle cells produce collagen and other reinforcement molecules, providing optimum stability and tone to the blood vessel wall. Long term deficiency of vitamins and other essential nutrients in millions of vascular wall cells impairs the function of the blood vessel walls.

Consequently, blood pressure increases, as does the development of fatty deposits, which in turn leads to heart attacks and strokes.

In the Harvard Nurses Study of 85,000 nurses, researchers from the School of Public Health found that women who had a vitamin C intake of more than 360 milligrams a day from diet and supplements had nearly a 30 percent reduction in their risk of heart disease.

Yet, *The Institute of Medicine* recommends a dietary allowance (RDA) of 90 mgs. for men and 75 mgs. for women of vitamin C per day. This recommendation will barely keep most consumers from getting scurvy, a wasting disease that leads to weakness of skin, gums and blood vessels. Insufficient vitamin C also leads to reduced ability to fight disease and premature death. According to the Pauling/Rath unified theory, both elevated homocysteine and oxidized cholesterol are symptoms of scurvy also.

Recommended Dietary Allowances (RDAs) for vitamins and minerals have been prepared by the Food and Nutrition Board of the National Research Council since 1941. These guidelines were originally developed to reduce the rates of severe nutritional deficiency diseases such as scurvy, pellagra (deficiency of niacin) and beriberi (deficiency of vitamin B1). RDAs were designed to serve as the basis for evaluating the adequacy of diets of groups of people, not individuals. Individuals are different and have varying nutritional needs. As stated by the Food and Nutrition Board *"Individuals with special nutritional needs are not covered by the RDAs."*

Jonathan V. Wright, M.D., editor in chief for *Nutrition & Healing*, suggests that most adults need 3 to 6 grams of vitamin C (3,000 to 6,000 milligrams) daily. When illness occurs, the amount should increase quite significantly. Because vitamin C is water-soluble and rapidly used by our bodies, it's best to consume it in equally divided amounts throughout the day.

Even with this information, the debate looms in scientific circles and critics continue to discredit the use of vitamin C. After the many years of research conducted by Dr. Linus Pauling and Matthias Rath, M.D., Roger J. Williams, Ph.D. and other scientists, medical schools, the pharmaceutical giants and the U.S. Government have ignored the benefits that large amounts of vitamin C and amino acids provide in relation to heart disease.

We know there is a very weak relationship between dietary cholesterol, blood cholesterol and the risk for heart disease. Yet, elevated levels of $Lp(a)$ are frequently overlooked by traditional medicine as a cause of heart disease. It is something that physicians need to consider when there is a clinical indication of heart disease.

Perhaps the reason why they overlook this theory is because there is no drug therapy for it (yet). Only vitamin C and lysine and proline can lower $Lp(a)$. I'm sure, in time, pharmaceutical companies will get wind of this and develop a drug that will not be nearly as safe as the natural supplements.

LYCOPENE

Lycopene has recently been studied in female subjects. Its benefits in lowering the risk of heart disease have been proven for both men and women. Lycopene is a carotenoid found primarily in tomatoes and, in lower concentrations, in watermelon, guava, rosehip, and red grapefruit. Lycopene has also been linked with reduced risk for prostate cancer, which is probably the main reason the recommendations for lycopene have been geared more toward men. Some preliminary research is showing, however, that it may also protect against breast cancer and cervical dysplasia, a precancerous condition in women. This new lycopene information is good news regarding its health benefits for men and women.

Coenzyme Q10 (CoQ10) Again

We are hearing quite a lot about CoQ10 these days and its effects on heart disease. More importantly, anyone taking statin drugs needs to be aware that these drugs deplete the production of CoQ10 in the body. CoQ10 deficiency can seriously affect the heart.

An essential component of the mitochondria, CoQ10 is the powerhouse of the cells. CoQ10 is involved in the manufacture of ATP, the energy currency of all body processes. It works similarly to a car's spark plugs. Without the spark, the car cannot run; so, too, CoQ10 is required for the human body to function. Research has shown that this super-antioxidant fuels cellular energy production and repairs free-radical damage to the heart muscle.

As we age, the levels of CoQ10 have been known to decline. This can also be due to nutritional deficiencies. Meat, poultry and fish provide the majority of dietary CoQ10; however, very little is obtained from food sources.

CoQ10 improves the function of the heart by improving energy production in the heart muscle and by acting as an antioxidant. Biopsy results from heart tissue in patients with various cardiovascular diseases showed a CoQ10 deficiency in 50-75 percent of cases.

Correction of a CoQ10 deficiency can often produce dramatic clinical results in patients with any kind of heart disease. Some practitioners recommend taking one milligram of CoQ10 for every pound of body weight. For instance, a 150 pound person would take 150 mg of CoQ10 each day. For conditions such as high blood pressure, mitral valve prolapse, angina and arrhythmia, 120-240 mgs. daily are recommended.

For people with serious heart problems, such as advanced congestive heart failure, doses as high as 300 to 400 mg per day are recommended.

Since CoQ10 is safe, find a practitioner who will work with you and who is familiar with this supplement and its benefits. There have been no adverse effects reported due to the use of CoQ10. If anything, the use of this great powerhouse has been shown to counteract some of the adverse effects of drugs. Once again the benefits outweigh the risks, just as Mother Nature intended.

The Bottom Line

As we have learned, heart disease is preventable. Unhealthy lifestyle behaviors are contributing factors in approximately 85 percent of those diagnosed with heart disease. It is much easier to prevent this condition than to treat it, thereby also preventing the costs and emotional trauma associated with treatment.

It's refreshing to know that a growing number of physicians are recognizing the benefits of positive lifestyle choices and find that this approach to treatment is as effective, if not more effective, than heart surgery. Do not be lured into surgery without knowing all the details and without doing your research. Think long and hard; re-read the topic about surgery in this chapter.

Although not mentioned in detail, the benefits of exercise are part and parcel to the lifestyle regime that needs to be incorporated into daily living. A simple 20-30 minute daily walk outdoors can make all the difference in the world regarding heart health.

I will end this chapter with several, heart-healthy tips for women and their families:

- Never smoke
- Exercise regularly

- Eat a nutritious, prudent diet that includes wholesome foods
- Find time to relax and manage stress
- Get at least 15-20 minutes of direct sunlight every day. **heart attacks are most common in the parts of the world that have the least sunshine.
- Avoid sugars, refined starches, or anything artificial
- Eat lots of fresh vegetables and fruits
- Use butter and olive oil instead of margarine
- Consume eggs, nuts and seeds, and avocados
- Sleep at least 7 hours/day (sleep deprivation manifests into other illnesses and diseases)
- If you consume alcohol, do so in moderation. Consider the benefits of red wine.
- Shop the periphery of the grocery stores where most of the whole foods are found
- Buy organic

If you are ever in a position when you are alone and feel that you may be experiencing a heart attack, here is some critical information that may save your life. Without assistance, a person whose heart stops beating properly and who begins to feel faint, has only about 10 seconds left before losing consciousness. You can help yourself.

This method has been used for years in cardiac catheter labs when people develop ventricular arrhythmias (abnormal heart rhythms).

- The victims can help themselves first by coughing repeatedly and very vigorously.
- A deep breath should be taken before each cough, and the cough must be deep and prolonged as when producing phlegm from deep inside the chest.

- This cough and a breath must be repeated about every two seconds without let up until help arrives or until the heart feels like it is beating normally again.

This works because the deep breaths move oxygen into the lungs; coughing squeezes the heart and keeps the blood circulating. The squeezing pressure on the heart also helps it regain normal rhythm. The heart attack victim can then get to a phone and, between breaths, call for help.

Share this information with everyone you can. And finally, remember, if you think you *are* having a heart attack, call your emergency medical system or 911 immediately. This suggestion is designed to give you the time you need to call for help: **IT IS NOT A SUBSTITUTE FOR PROFESSIONAL MEDICAL HELP.**

*"There are two ways to be fooled. One is to believe
what isn't true; the other is to refuse to believe
what is true."*
— *Soren Kierkegaard*

THE FINAL ANALYSIS...

PUTTING IT ALL INTO PERSPECTIVE

PEOPLE ARE TURNING AWAY FROM modern medicine, not
because it is ineffective, but because it is inhumane. This is quite
a profound statement, expressed at the London Medical Society
in May 1999. Although I agree that modern medicine is inhumane in several aspects, I do believe women are turning away
from modern medicine for other reasons.

Modern medicine, in many cases, has been essentially ineffective and painful due to its paradigm of treating and suppressing
symptoms without regard to safety and healing.

Learning about a variety of options and safer alternatives,
as presented in previous chapters, is driving the impetus for
women to begin to ask questions. There are always alternative
solutions to healthcare issues and problems, alternative solutions that should be wisely explored before more invasive
approaches are implemented. Use your intuition.

A friend of our family told me, after reading, experimenting
and achieving great results due to some lifestyle changes, that
he and his wife have adopted the *MEDS* tradition for their family,

a tradition that is becoming the cornerstone of their life:

Meditation/prayer – Exercise – Diet/nutrition – Sleep/rest.

They are learning that conventional methods of preventing and managing illness and disease through drugs are *not* the answer.

Massive and sophisticated marketing campaigns do not make drugs harmless, as I have indicated throughout these chapters. After so many years of negative messages and half-truths, it takes time, education and a truthful consistent message to create the breakthrough. Introducing synthetic and artificial substances into the body disturbs other functions of the body and creates imbalance. I have discussed the importance of balance and how it plays a major role in achieving good health and healing. Always consider the risk benefit ratio.

*B*y now you should understand that drugs do not prevent disease, choices do. Thomas Jefferson was way ahead of his time when he said, *"If people let the government decide what foods they eat and what medicines they take, their bodies will soon be in a sorry state, as are the souls who live under tyranny."*

Is this what we are experiencing today? I have shared with you personal stories, stories from clients and the conflicting information that is reported on a daily basis, information that continues to confuse women to the point of incomprehensible frustration. I have provided a point/counterpoint snapshot of some of the most devastating chronic illnesses and conditions that women suffer from today.

To augment this information, I will close with a few more facts, tips, guidelines and suggestions. I cannot guarantee that they will help you live longer, but they will certainly go a long way toward enhancing your quality of life. With a little dedication and knowledge, you too, can enjoy the rewards of good health.

JUST GO NATURAL

As I've said all along, an informed consumer is a better consumer. Going natural will require you to read labels and learn how to avoid toxic ingredients to which we are exposed on a daily basis.

Just as consuming artificial foods and chemicals will wreak havoc on our bodies, so too will exposure to other products we buy at the grocery store, such as insect repellents, cleaners, cosmetics, plastics and over-the-counter drugs.

Even though a product is marketed as "natural" it may contain additional ingredients that are not. Some companies label their products as "natural" but this may not mean 100 percent. Be sure to read the labels thoroughly.

AVOIDING THE DANGERS IN YOUR HOME

Researchers found that Parkinson's disease is directly linked to exposure to pesticides. People exposed to high levels of pesticides found in the home carry the highest risk of developing the disease by 70 percent. Parkinson's disease was unheard of 200 years ago. It has now become the second most common degenerative nerve disease.

Another study linked the use of herbicides and pesticides in California to an increased risk of Parkinson's disease. California uses over 250 million pounds of pesticides annually, roughly one-fourth of all the pesticides used in the United States. Researchers found that the incidence of Parkinson's was significantly greater in those agricultural counties where the chemicals were being used

Exposure to organophosphates, the active compounds in

pesticides like Dursban, Diazinon, and Malathion, inhibit the formation of the cholinesterase enzyme in the nervous system that kills insects. Similarly, this process occurs in humans, too, whereby the transmission of nerve impulses is blocked. It's the constant exposure to these chemicals that increases your risk of developing serious diseases and conditions. Oftentimes, symptoms are delayed, not showing up for years. Err on the side of caution. It is much safer to avoid toxic chemicals now than to guess whether or not exposure to them will cause serious long term effects.

Do not use any insecticides, herbicides or fungicides in your home. Avoid using a bug service on a monthly or yearly basis. Household paints, thinners, mineral spirits, motor oils or any petroleum products are dangerous. It is imperative to protect yourself when using these products, if you must use them at all. Wear gloves and long sleeves and avoid skin contact. Always use these chemicals in an open area with fresh air. Clean up is vitally important, as important as disposing of the containers. Read directions thoroughly.

ALTERNATIVES TO PESTICIDES, COMMERCIAL CLEANERS, AND OTHER HOUSEHOLD PRODUCTS

BRONNER'S PURE-CASTILE PEPPERMINT SOAP

Mix five drops of liquid soap to one quart of water and spray away. This is a safe and effective alternative for use in the garden to eliminate pests. This liquid soap can be found in local health food stores. It can be used for everything from ants to aphids to whiteflies and, believe it or not, for bathing as well. A four to five dollar bottle will last a long time. Liquid dishwashing soap is also effective as a plant spray.

Mix (1T) of liquid dishwashing soap in two cups of water. Apply to effected plants using a spray bottle. Make sure you saturate the undersides of the leaves. You may have to repeat this application several times. This is a non-toxic treatment that will not harm the plants, the kids or the animals.

BORIC ACID.

To get rid of some of the creepier bugs in nature, such as fleas, termites, and cockroaches, try the old standby, boric acid. It was used years ago for everything, including eyewashes. Even today, people will use it as a wound cleanser for their dogs and cats. It is sold in pet stores and garden shops. Sprinkle this powder around the edges of rooms and underneath sinks where cockroaches enter regularly. It can be dusted in carpets and furniture and then vacuumed up. The little bit that cannot be picked up by the vacuum will remain and kill the intruders. It can also be sprinkled under houses for termites. Chrysanthemum oil can also be used to rid a home of pesky bugs.

DIATOMACEOUS EARTH.

This is for indoor use to control cockroaches, ants, earwigs, silverfish, crickets, millipedes, and centipedes. Lightly coat a thin layer of dust in the areas where these pests are found or may hide, such as cracks and crevices, behind and beneath stoves, refrigerators, sinks, cabinets, garbage cans, around pipes and drains, window frames, and in attics and basements. Hit insects directly when possible. Repeat as necessary. *Do not* use the diatomaceous earth product used for swimming pools.

POISON AND MOUSETRAP SUBSTITUTES.

Instead of buying mousetraps and poison bait for rodents or insects, stuff steel wool into the holes around the plumbing pipes under the sinks in your bathrooms and kitchen to keep the critters out.

JET DRY SUBSTITUTE.

Instead of spending money for a commercial rinse agent like Jet Dry for your dishwasher, use plain white vinegar. You only need to fill the dispenser every few weeks. Your glassware will sparkle, remain spot-free and the inside of the dishwasher will remain clean.

OVEN CLEANER THE NON-TOXIC WAY.

Most commercial oven cleaners have a very strong and lingering smell. For a fresher approach, add one teaspoon (1tsp) each of liquid soap, lemon juice, vinegar and borax to one quart of warm water. Apply liberally to the inside of the oven and allow it to sit for at least 30 minutes. Then scrub.

Vinegar can be an effective alternative to conventional herbicides for organic farmers and gardeners, say scientists from the Agriculture Department.

Household vinegar contains about 5 percent acetic acid, the ingredient that kills weeds, according to Jay Radhakrishnan, agronomist. Concentrations of five to ten percent will kill all weeds during the first two weeks of their life. I can attest to this. I use vinegar on my weeds in the yard all the time. It takes them from a few days to a week to die, but it is very effective. Be sure to spray the leaves on the weeds well. The leaves absorb the vinegar down to the root that causes the weed to die. Spot spraying of corn fields with a 20 percent concentration of acetic acid kills 80 to 100 percent of weeds without harming the corn.

Vinegar is also a deterrent to mold and fungus. Over time, air conditioning units and their vents and returns build up mold. During maintenance checks, technicians will spray a fruity chemical to disguise the smell that goes away in a short period of time. However, in the meantime, this chemical has been dispersed throughout the house through the air conditioning system.

Instead, put non-diluted vinegar in a spray bottle and spray directly into all of your return air vents on a regular basis to avoid a mold buildup. You may find this will decrease allergies and runny noses over time. This is an especially good idea when moving into a new house. It will prevent mold from ever building up.

BIOPESTICIDES

Biopesticides (also known as biological pesticides) are certain types of pesticides derived from such natural materials as plants, bacteria, and certain minerals. For example, garlic, mint, and baking soda all have pesticidal applications and are considered biopesticides. At the end of 1998, there were approximately 175 registered biopesticide active ingredients and 700 products.

To learn more about how to rid your home of critters, insects and other annoying bugs by using non-toxic approaches, see *Resources* in the back of this book, or visit the EPA website under "Google" search and type in biopesticides.

Do not use petro-chemically based perfumed air fresheners or aerosol cans, plug-ins and other scented items at home or in the car. Many consumers think the lemon scents and strawberry scents are nice, but they are chemicals that are actually disguising smells.

Walk into a hotel room sometime and you will really get a strong whiff of these chemicals. Using vinegar and baking soda will take care of unsightly odors and is safer, not only for the person cleaning but for everyone. It amazes me that large hotels don't use these cleaners, because they are much less expensive and far safer.

Some consumers have become so sensitive to these odors in hotels that they are not only asking for smoke-free rooms, but for odor-free rooms as well. The next time you travel, request a room that has not been deodorized by chemicals.

These are just a few of many safe, economical and viable alternatives that should be introduced into your home to decrease your exposure to potentially toxic chemicals.

PLASTICS

Although economical and convenient, there has been a great deal of concern and research around the dangers of plastics in our environment over the past 50 years. Recently, an article was published about the dangers of microwaving in plastic containers and storing foods in plastics such as water, soda pop and other liquids. To address the rumor mill, Ralph Halden, PhD, PE, assistant professor in the Department of Environmental Health Sciences and the Center for Water and Health at the Johns Hopkins Bloomberg School of Public Health, provided some insight.

Dioxins are organic environmental pollutants that are known to be the most toxic compounds made by mankind. Exposure to these dioxins can disrupt reproductive activity in humans and can cause developmental effects, liver damage and cancer.

Phthalates, sometimes added to plastics to make them flexible and less brittle, are environmental contaminants that can exhibit hormone-like behavior by acting as endocrine disruptors in humans and animals. If you heat up plastics, you could increase the leaching of phthalates from the containers into water and food.

Now let's apply logic. When you heat something you increase the likelihood of chemicals leaching out. Chemicals can be released from plastic packaging materials like the kinds used in some microwave meals. A straw placed into a boiling cup of hot tea or coffee, or plastic wrap on top of food in the microwave, is creating an extraction of chemicals which can infiltrate into the food. This is done in laboratories all the time for scientific analysis of materials.

Since we know that plastics are made of toxic materials that, when heated, leach out, it would be wise to avoid the use of plastics when cooking or covering hot foods. If you are using plastic utensils, follow the directions and only use plastics that are specifically meant for cooking. Stainless steel utensils are preferable. Your best bet is to use inert containers, such as those made of glass or stainless steel.

Prior to the ubiquitous use of plastics in our environment, glass was used almost exclusively. Think about how our milk, sodas and other liquids used to be stored. More progressive organic packaging is beginning to move back to the basics of glass for storage. It's the safest thus far.

Even though scientists say that a miniscule amount of chemical contaminants are present in these containers, I suggest to err on the side of caution and avoid using these containers. Regarding bottled water, we are not only concerned about the plastics, but we are also suspicious of the quality of the water.

You will be better served to install a water system in your home rather than to buy cases of bottled water. No one knows how long these cases of water may be sitting on docks or in trucks in hot weather. Furthermore, in the long run, it is more economical and convenient. And if you must take water along with you as you travel, at least you know where your water is coming from, even if you use a plastic container for temporary storage.

As discussed in earlier chapters, it's the cumulative effect that is dangerous and it's the dosage of the chemical that makes it poison.

COSMETICS AND PERSONAL HYGIENE

Many chemicals that are classified as hazardous substances are in the beauty products we use on a daily basis. Many of them contain petroleum derivatives that can cause skin irritation and other problems. Even though you may not have had any negative reactions using these ingredients, why expose yourself to known carcinogens and unnecessary chemicals when there are so many natural products that are much safer and gentler for the skin? Just as I strongly recommend avoiding foods that contain preservatives, dyes and colors, so, too, should you avoid these ingredients in cosmetics.

Valerie Gennari Cooksley, R.N., cofounder of the Institute of Integrative Aromatherapy has this to say about chemicals in cosmetics: *"Using toxic chemical-laden body care products can, over time, block the body's elimination pathways. Nature provides ways to get rid of waste from the body through the lungs, kidneys, bowels, and the skin. But if these elimination pathways become clogged or backed up, the body will not function properly, health will be diminished, and conditions like environmental illness can develop."*

It's the constant exposure of chemicals being introduced into our bodies daily that creates potential health risks. If you are suffering from any chronic illnesses or diseases, evaluate your use of cosmetics. Obviously, the more toxic the ingredients the product contains, the worse it is.

Most women do not think exposure to chemicals through their cosmetics can affect their health, but science tells us otherwise. The beauty of "natural" products is that they are free from harsh chemicals that can cause severe damage.

Listed below are some of the ingredients you should avoid:

- Acetone – an eye and lung irritant found in nail polish, nail polish removers and astringents. It can cause central nervous system disorders.
- BHA and BHT – preservatives.
- DEA – a harmful cancer-causing chemical.
- Diazolodinyl Urea – used as a pesticide.

- Imidazolidinyl Urea and Diazolidinyl Urea – can cause contact dermatitis according to the American Academy of Dermatology.
- Methyl, Propyl, Butyl and Ethyl Paraben (parabens) – preservatives to extend shelf life of products that can cause allergic reactions and skin rashes and may be absorbed as estrogenic in the body.
- Parabens – synthetic preservative to extend shelf life of a product. Some researchers are suggesting they are xenoestrogens that have an estrogenic effect on the body.
- Petrolatum – mineral oil jelly produced from by-products of petroleum.
- Phthalates – industrial chemicals used as plastic softeners or solvents are endocrine disrupters known to cause tumors in animals or disrupt the hormone activity of humans.
- Propylene Glycol (PEG) – known to cause allergic and toxic reactions.
- PVP/VA Copolymer – widely used in hairsprays and gels. These are petroleum derivatives found to be toxic when inhaled.
- Sodium Lauryl Sulfate – detergents that can cause eye irritations, skin rashes, hair loss, and other allergic reactions. Often advertised as "comes from coconut."
- Synthetic Colors – FD&C, D&C followed by a color or number. They contain cancer causing agents.
- Synthetic Fragrances – avoid anything with a label that contains them.

Instead of the ingredients listed above, look for products that contain botanicals, essential oils, coconut oil, herbs, vitamins, plant oils and other vegetable-based ingredients. Look for antioxidants such as grapeseed oils, almond, apricot, olive and jojoba oils that nourish and protect the skin. Lavender, tea tree, sodium bicarbonate (baking soda) also keep the skin clean.

Beauty products that contain herbs, vitamins or other nutrients can be much more beneficial. Always read labels. The first few ingredients that appear on the product contain the greatest concentration in the product.

Be wise and prudent, and search out products that are safe. Look under *Resources* listed in the back of the book to help you search out these fine products.

Is the Nail Polish Industry in Denial?

A dear friend, who is a professional career woman and mother of two, says she must keep her nails looking good because when she does business presentations, she wants to look attractive and more professional. I'm sure there are many women who echo her sentiments.

Don't tell a woman that painting her nails can be toxic. Even amid the health concerns, she will turn the other way and take her chances anyway.

According to the Cosmetics Toiletry and Fragrance association trade group, the nail polish industry has become valued as a $650 million industry with fancy nails that are painted with scenery and other depictions of everything from animals to snowflakes. If you don't believe me regarding the toxicity from this industry, try walking into a beauty salon without having to take a second breath. It can be nauseating because the chemicals are so strong.

Not only do these chemicals smell nasty, but the damage they do to the nail bed is frightening, as is the immediate absorption into your body. Natural nails become discolored and lose their natural beauty. This is one reason why once women begin to get their nails painted, they must always have them painted because their nails turn so unsightly. Another coat of paint covers up what is really going on underneath.

NAIL POLISH MAKERS TAKING A (HESITANT) TURN

Phthalates, (pronounced THA-layts) are being aggressively removed from the European cosmetic markets. Beginning in September 2004, di-n-butyl phthalate (DBP) and di (2ethyl-hexyl) phthalate (DEHP) were banned from the cosmetic marketplace.

Although the U.S. industry does not believe there is a health risk, two major cosmetic companies are phasing out the use of these volatile chemicals that are known to be toxic, especially to women in their childbearing years. Procter & Gamble and Estee Lauder companies are planning to reformulate their products to remove these chemicals. These chemicals are toxic when you breathe them and when you put them on your nails.

Even though the National Toxicology Program, a division of the Department of Health and Human Services (DHHS), acknowledges the risks shown in lab studies, these companies will not acknowledge that the drive to remove these chemicals is due to toxicity and dangers. This is interesting. After all, if there was no validity to this statement, there is no way companies would spend thousands of dollars to reformulate just for the sake of reformulating.

DHHS does not believe the U.S. population has been exposed to DBP levels too high for immediate concern, yet there is concern in the air. I do not believe them. Gerald McEwan, vice president for science at the Washington-based trade group, quotes, *"This is more a matter of politics than of science."* Have we heard this before?

A San Francisco-based Breast Cancer Fund group has requested that several manufacturers reformulate their products. Evidently the pressure from these groups is forcing these companies to change. In California, DBP and DEHP are already on a list of potential carcinogenic or reproductive toxins.

Even though companies may be removing these chemicals due to outside pressure, don't think for a moment that their products are any safer. They still contain other unwelcome ingredients, such as acetates, chemical dyes, formaldehyde and toluene.

Formaldehyde may temporarily harden nails, but ends up dehydrating the nail. This makes the nail bed more susceptible to becoming brittle, chipped and splitting. Acetone is terribly drying and lifts the oils right out of the nails, according to Dr. Bruce Katz, dermatologist and director of the JUVA skin and laser center in New York.

NAIL POLISH FOR THE PURIST

Evidently, some companies are taking this threat of dangerous chemicals more seriously than others. Companies are now creating new solvent-free nail polishes. Honeybee Gardens has created a mineral and water based product that can be removed with rubbing alcohol or grain alcohol. They also have a peel-off version that only lasts about 2 days, but requires no remover.

Acquarella Water Colors includes a line of nail conditioner, polish remover, moisture and polishes. Sante Kosmetiks Nail Enamels is a product line free of phthalates and synthetic preservatives or fragrances. These natural products do not last as long as the industrial strength common nail polishes, but you will be able to breathe easier and introduce them to your daughters without fear of toxicity.

THE PARCELLS OXYGEN SOAK

Purchasing organic foods may not be affordable for some folks, yet the concern of toxicity in the form of insecticides, pesticides and other chemicals is a very real concern.

There is an old remedy that only costs pennies that has been reported as being extremely effective in removing the toxins from foods. The Parcells Oxygen Soak method was developed by Hazel Parcells, ND, in the 1950s and is currently registered with the Smithsonian Institution under *"Simplified Kitchen Chemistry"*. It is used around the world with great success, having been adopted by health departments of many governments.

Dr. Parcells conducted an experiment at Sierra State University in California with shriveled, discolored lemons meant for the compost pile. She placed them in a sink full of water into which she put a small amount of bleach. Within one-half hour the lemons had taken on a fresh appearance and the room smelled of fragrant lemon.

Dr. Parcells pulled them out, separated them in pieces and placed them in a freezer. They were tested for freshness and nutritional value over 3 years. Through the third year they retained their freshness, moisture, tartness and rivaled fresh lemons, even in nutritional value. Thus began Dr. Parcell's pursuit of researching ways to restore vitality to foods.

I know you may be concerned about the use of bleach, since we all know how toxic bleach can be, however, the amount of bleach used is what makes the difference. Just like alcohol: A shot may not kill you, but a bottle will.

Household bleach is not chlorine like you put in a swimming pool. In fact, it's no more chlorine than common table salt is (sodium chloride). Chlorine is used in the making of household bleach, but the end product contains no free chlorine. Bleach is produced by combining chlorine and caustic soda (sodium hydroxide). When the two products are combined, they convert into sodium hypochlorite, the active ingredient in household bleach. The Clorox® bottle contains 5.25 percent solution of sodium hypochlorite and water.

Soaking Instructions

Use 1 teaspoon of Clorox® bleach to 1 gallon of water. Foods should be separated into the following categories:

VEGETABLES

Leafy vegetables	5-10 minutes
Root and heavy fiber vegetables	10-15 minutes

FRUITS

Thin-skinned fruits, such as berries	5 minutes
Medium-skinned fruits like peaches, apricots and plums	10 minutes
Thick-skinned fruits like apples	10-15 minutes
Citrus fruits and bananas	15 minutes

EGGS	20-30 minutes

MEATS

Meats/poultry per pound (thawed),	10 minutes
frozen	15-20 minutes

Do not use more than 1 teaspoon of bleach per gallon of water and do not soak the food any longer than suggested. The last part of the directions is equally important. Remove the food and place it in a gallon or more of fresh water to rinse for 5-10 minutes. This step introduces a flood of new oxygen into the food. Dry the food well before storage.

This process removes any type of fungus, bacteria or other substances that may be toxic. I soak most of my foods and even some of my organic produce that is covered in dirt. Use only original Clorox®, not the scented formulas.

Dry Cleaning Leaves Serious Residues

There are some risks in life we are unable to avoid because we do not live in a perfect world. But we should take charge over the things we can control.

Most women don't think twice about traipsing to the dry cleaners on a weekly basis to get their clothes cleaned. In fact, dry cleaning services have popped up everywhere across the nation due to consumer demand.

Once again, there are some serious consequences to dry cleaning, long term, that the average person never thinks about. Perchloroethylene (Perc) is a chlorinated hydrocarbon that was originally developed as a metal degreaser for airplane parts. It is also a suspected endocrine disrupter, meaning it is a chemical that may confuse the body into thinking it is estrogen. More than 34,000 dry cleaners use 57 million pounds of Perc each year.

A 1994 study by the National Institute for Occupational Safety and Health found that dry cleaning workers had seven times the average rate of esophageal cancer and twice the rate of bladder cancer. A study published in the February 2001 issue of the *American Journal of Industrial Medicine* found excessive deaths among 1,708 dry cleaning workers exposed to Perc for at least a year.

People living near dry cleaners may be exposed to potentially high levels of Perc if vapors move up through apartment buildings or office buildings. New York recently forced dry cleaning shops in residential buildings to meet strict new standards for equipment, pollution prevention and ventilation.

IF YOU MUST DRY CLEAN

If you must dry clean, there are a few simple measures to employ. Immediately remove the plastic covering the clothes and let the clothes hang outside or in the garage to air out for 12–24 hours. This enables the fumes to be released outside your home. Dry clean suits, coats and jackets less frequently. Usually it's only the underarms that need attention versus the entire fabric.

Clothing that is labeled "dry clean only" or "dry cleaning recommended" can often be washed in a delicate cycle in the washing machine. (We are trying to convince our daughter of this to help her save hundreds of dollars per year she spends on dry cleaning). Silks, wools, and rayon in particular can be washed on gentle or by hand, but clothing that is lined should probably be dry cleaned as recommended.

Use delicate soaps such as the ones available in health food stores or Dr. Bronner's baby liquid castile soap. Lay wools flat on a towel and *do not* wring or twist out. Try to form the garment to the correct size before it dries.

Spot cleaning with white vinegar is an option also. Do not do this on rayon, however. It is a very delicate fabric and could stain.

Wet Cleaning is becoming more popular today. It is not less expensive than dry cleaning, but the dry cleaning chemicals will be avoided. You can check out more information in the *Resource* section at the back of this book.

Your Healing Path

Hopefully, you have learned about some breakthroughs in natural approaches to health and healing in this book and about behaviors that will lead you toward optimal health. It's a journey.

Some folks tell me I am wasting my time trying to teach consumers about natural approaches to healthy living and healing. They tell me that there are very few people who will change their behavior based on what I report and say.

I look at it from a different perspective. Just like a farmer who plants thousands of seeds, many are wasted in the process for unknown reasons. However, no matter the waste, the seeds that do find fertile soil and germinate into maturity will produce a crop a hundred times more than what was wasted.

As the farmer does not stop planting because every grain

planted does not grow, nor will I stop teaching and educating just because every woman does not hear my message. If my message is not well received, I will move on so as not to get caught up in useless arguments and volatile rhetoric.

If we all applied the same pessimistic attitude as some, nothing would get done, nor would we change or grow. I know this from professional experience with my clients.

Those who are optimistic, listen and take action always touch others abundantly and experience a far greater benefit beyond the small seeds of knowledge I have planted.

REFERENCES

INTRODUCTION

1 "Drug Company Influence on Medical Education in USA," editorial, *Lancet* 356: 781,2000. [Medline]
2 Ralph W. Moss Reports, *Cancer Decisions*, June 2003.
3 *Wall Street Journal*, August, 2003.
4 *Health Affairs*, 2003.
5 Vioxx Lawsuits may focus on FDA Warning in 2001, *Wall Street Journal*, October 5, 2004.

CHAPTER 1: A TIME FOR CHANGE

1 Starfield, B., Is U.S. Health Really the Best in the World? *JAMA* 284:483-488, 2000.
2 *Economist*, June 24, 2000.
3 *American College of Sports Medicine, Health and Fitness Journal* November/December 2003.
4 McGinnis, J.M. and W.H. Foege. Actual Causes of Death in the U.S. *JAMA* 270:2207-2212, 1993.
5 *Health Affairs*, May 4, 2004.
6 Starfield, B., M.D., MPH, Medical Errors – A Leading Cause of Death, *JAMA* July 26, 2000, Vol 284, No 4.
7 Nuland, S.B. *Whoops!* The New York Review of Books, July 18, 2002;10-13.

CHAPTER 2: HORMONE REPLACEMENT THERAPY (HRT) . . . TRUTH VERSUS HALF-TRUTHS

1 Rodriguez, C., Calle, E.E., Coates, R. J., Miracle-McMahill, H. L., Thun, M. J., Heath, C.W. Jr. Estrogen replacement therapy and fatal ovarian cancer. *Am J Epidemiol* 1995;141:828-835.
2 Challem, Jack "Medicalizing Life," Newswire, The Nutrition

Reporter, *Let's Live Magazine*, Sept. 2002.

3   Zhand, F., et al. The major metabolite of equilin, 4-hydroxye-quilin,autoxidizes to an opquinone which isomerizes to the potent cytotoxin 4-hydroxequilenin-o-quinine. *Chem Res Toxicol* 1999 Feb; 12 (2):204-13.

4   Vaughan, Paul. *The Pill on Trial*. London: Weidenfeld and Nicolson, 1970:25.

5   Paul, C., et al. Depot medroxyprogesterone (Depo-Provera) and risk of breast cancer. *Br Med J* 1989;299:759.

6   Lee, John R., *What Your Doctor May Not Tell You About Menopause*, 1996.

7   Coney, Sandra. *The Menopause Industry*. Alameda, CA: Hunter House, 1994.

8   *Consumer Reports* Licit and Illicit Drugs: The Consumer's Union Report on Narcotics, Stimulants, Depressants, Inhalants, Hallucinogens, and Marijuana, Including Caffeine, Nicotine, and Alcohol (Boston: Little, Brown, 1973).

9   Shankar, Vedantam, "FDA Study Confirms Antidepressant Risks", *Washington* Post, August 10, 2004.

10   *National Institute of Mental Health*, 2003.

11   "The Case for Hormone Therapy," *JAMA*, July 2002; 288:321-333.

12   Ibid.

13   Glass, Margery, M.D., St. Petersburg Times, *"Not by Hormones Alone,"* November, 2003.

14   Bergkvist, pg. 293 *NEJM* 3, Aug 89.

15   T.S. Wiley, Taguchi, J., M.D., Formby, B., Ph.D., *Sex, Lies and Menopause*, 2003.

16   Colbert, Don, M.D., *Toxic Relief*, 2001.

17   Ibid.

18   Beral, V.; Million Women Study Collaborators, Breast cancer and hormone-replacement therapy in the Million Women Study, *Lancet*. 2003 Oct 4;362(9390):1160.

19   Ibid.

20   Topical estrogen approved for treating hot flashes: lotion for short-term use only - *GynecologyOB/GYN News*, November 15, 2003.

21   *Canadian Cancer Society*, "New Recommendation about

Combined Hormone Replacement Therapy," January 8, 2004.

22 "National Use of Postmenopausal Hormone Therapy: Annual Trends and Response to Recent Evidence," *Fam Community Health*. 2003;26 (1) : 53-63.

23 *The People Pharmacy Guide to Home and Herbal Remedies* (St. Martin's Press) 2002.

CHAPTER 3: BALANCING HORMONES . . .
A SAFER AND GENTLER APPROACH

1 MR Publishing, Inc., *Cellular Health Communications*, Vol. 2, Number 1, 2003.

2 Lee, John R., M.D., Hanley, J, M.D. and Hopkins, V., *What Your Doctor May Not Tell You About Premenopause*, Warner Books, Inc., 1999.

3 J. Gregory,"Denaturation of the Folacin-binding Protein in Pasteurized Milk Products," *Journal of Nutrition* 112:7 (July 1982): 1329-1338.

4 Health Science Institute e-alert, Complex made Simple, HSI Research@healthiernews.com June 2003.

5 Colbert, Don, M.D., *Toxic Relief*, 2001.

6 MR Publishing, *Cellular Health Communications*, Vol. 2, Number 1, 2003.

7 Rath, Matthias, M.D., *Ten Years that Changed Medicine Forever*, 2001.

8 Rath, Matthias, M.D., *Why Animals Don't Get Heart Attacks . . . But People Do!*, 2000.

9 Bjelland, I., Tell GS, Vollset SE, Refsum H, Ueland PM, *Archives of General Psychiatry*, June, 2003;60(6)618-26. *British Med J*, 1998.

10 Sheffrey, Stephen, D.D.S, *Who's Kidding Who about Vitamin C*, 1998.

11. *http://www.hsibaltimore.com/ea2004/ea_040227.shtml*

12. Lark, Susan, M.D., *Dr. Lark's Guide To Optimal Health and Balance For Women*, Nutritional Supplementation, 2002, page. 9.

13. Mercola, Joseph, D.O., and Droege, R., *Want to Live Longer?* Eat More Flavonoids., 2004.

14. Ibid.

15 S. Weir Newmayer, AM, M.D., *The Human Body and its Care*, American Book Company, 1928.

16 Teitelbaum, J., M.D., Highly Effective Treatments for Pain and Fatigue, *Townsend Letter for Doctors and Patients*, June 2004 pg. 138.

17 *New York Times Magazine*, May 6, 2001.

18 Lark, Susan, M.D., *The Lark Letter*, September, 2003.

19 Walsh, Nancy, Studies find black cohosh eases menopause symptoms. *Family Practice News*. March, 2001.

20 Mauskop, A., Altura, B. T., Cracco, R. Q., Altura, B. M., Intravenous magnesium sulfate rapidly alleviates headaches of various types. *Headache* 36 (1996):154-60.

21 Asami, D. K., Hong, Y. J., Barrett, D. M., Mitchell, A. E. Comparison of the total phenolic and ascorbic acid content of freeze-dried and air-dried marionberry, strawberry, and corn grown using conventional, organic, and sustainable agricultural practices. *J Agric Food Chem*. 2003 Feb 26;51(5):1237-41.

22 Annual Meeting for the Society of Maternal-Fetal Medicine, February, 2003.

23 Lee, John R., M.D., *What Your Doctor May Not Tell You About Menopause*, 1996. pgs. 258-259.

24 Reprinted with permission from: *What Your Doctor May Not Tell You About Breast Cancer*, 2002, Lee, John R., M.D., Zava, D., Ph.D., and Hopkins, V.

25 Choe, J. K., Khan-Dawood, F. S., Dawood, M.Y. *Am J Obstet Gynecol* 1983 Nov.;147:557-562.

26 Harris B, Lovett L, Newcombe, R.G., Read, G.F., Walker, R., Riad-Fahmy, D. Maternity blues and major endocrine changes: Cardiff puerperal mood and hormone study II. *BMJ* 1994 Apr;308:949-953.

27 Lee, John R., M.D., Zava, D., Ph.D., Hopkins, V., *What Your Doctor May Not Tell You About Breast Cancer*, 2002.

CHAPTER 4: THE BREAST CANCER INDUSTRY . . . THE DARK SIDE OF HALF-TRUTHS

1 *American Cancer Society*, 2004.

2 Clifton Leaf, Why We're Losing the War on Cancer-and How to Win It, *Fortune*, March 2004.

3   *American Cancer Society*, 1999-2000.

4   *American Cancer Society, Cancer Facts and Figures 2003.*

5   *Alternative Therapies*, June 2004, Vol. 10, No. 3. pg. 83.

6   *Alternative Therapies*, Sept. 1997, Vol. 3, No. 5. pgs. 39-52.

7   Ibid. pg.45.

8   Begley, Sharon. Why targeted drugs to battle cancer fall short of promise. *Wall Street Journal, Science Journal*, Sept. 10, 2004.

9   *WHO Report:* www.who.int/mediacentre/releases /2003/pr27/en/

10 *Alternative Medicine*, Breast Cancer Awareness, Nov. 2001, pgs. 68-74.

11 *Z Magazine On-line*, October 2003 Volume 16 Number 10.

12 Abelson, Reed. Drug sales bring huge profits, and scrutiny to cancer doctors. *New York Times*. January 26, 2003, page A1. Cancer scare tactics: *New York Times* editorial, March 22, 2004.

13 T.S. Wiley, Taguchi, J., M.D., and Formby, B., Ph.D., *Sex, Lies, and Menopause*, 2003.

14 Love, Susan, M. Quoted by: Sharp N. The politics of breast cancer. *Nurs Manage* 1991; 22(9):24-28.

15 Dr. Susan Love's Breast Book. Reading, Mass: Addison-Wesley; 1990:212.

16 Sherrill Sellman, *"Hormone Heresy : What Women Must Know About Their Hormones"*, 1998.

17 Plotkin D., Good news and bad news about breast cancer. *The Atlantic Monthly*. June 1996.

18 Hellman, S., Harris, J. The appropriate breast cancer paradigm. *Cancer Res.* 1987; 47:341.

19 Institute of Medicine at the National Academies in Washington, June 2004.

20 *Journal of the National Cancer Institute* September 20, 2000; 92:1490-1499.

21 Bailar, J.C.,III "Mammagrapy-A Time for Caution." *JAMA* 237 (10) (1977): 997-998.

22 Lee, John R.,M.D., Zava, D., Ph.D., and Hopkins, V., *What Your Doctor May Not Tell You About Breast Cancer*, 2002.

23 Lark, Susan, M.D., *The Lark Letter*, May 2003, pg. 4.

24 Goldberg, Burton, What you're not being told about mammography, *Alternative Medicine*, Oct.23, 2000.

25 *Time Magazine,* "Rethinking Breast Cancer" with a subtitle "New detection techniques and treatments are exciting-and confusing. A guide to saving lives." February 18, 2002 Vol. 159 No. 7.

26 U.S. Preventive Services Task Force, 2002.

27 Mary S. Wolff and others, "Blood Levels of Organochlorine Residues and Risk of Breast Cancer," *Journal Of The National Cancer Institute* Vol. 85 April 21, 1993, pgs. 648-652.

28 Conversations with Mitchell Gaynor, M.D., *Alternative Therapies,* May/June 2004, Vol. 10, No. 3.

29 Harriet Beinfield, Lac, and Malcolm S. Beinfield, M.D., FACS, Revisiting Accepted Wisdom in the Management of Breast Cancer, *Alternative Therapies,* Sept. 1997, Vol. 3, No. 5.

30 Ibid. pgs. 43-52.

31 Henderson, B. E., Ross. R., Bernstein, L. Estrogen is a cause of human cancer: The Richard and Hilda Rosenthal Foundation Award Lecture. *Cancer Research* 1988;48:246-53.

32 Trudy L. Bush, Ph. D, MHS; Maura K. Whiteman, *JAMA,* June 9, 1999;281:2091-2097, 2140-2141.

33 Hufford, D. J., Ph. D, Cultural Diversity, Folk Medicine, and Alternative Medicine, *Alternative Therapies,* July 1997, Vol. 3, No. 4, pgs.79-80.

34 Ibid. pg. 28.

CHAPTER 5: BREAST CANCER PREVENTION

1 *WHO Report:* www.who.int/mediacentre/releases /2003/pr27/en/

2 *Alternative Therapies in Health and Medicine.* 1996;2(6):32-38.

3 Murray, Michael T., N.D., Pizzorno, J.E., N.D., *Encyclopedia of Natural Medicine, Revised 2nd Edition,* 1998.

4 *Cancer Res* 2000;60(20):5635-39.

5 Lee, John R., M.D., Zava, D., PhD., Hopkins, V., *What Your Doctor May Not Tell You About Breast Cancer,* 2002.

6 *Prog Clin Biol Res* 1996;394:211-53.

7 LeMaitre, G. D. *How to Choose a Good Doctor.* Andover, Mass: Andover Publishing Group; 1979.

8 Mohr, P. E., et al. Serum progesterone and prognosis in operable breast cancer, *Br. J. Cancer,* 1996, Jun; 73 (12) 1552-1555.

9   Cowan LD et al. Breast cancer incidence in women with a history of progesterone deficiency, *American Journal of Epidemiology,* *1981; 114: 209-17.*

10 K. J. Chang, T.T.Y. Lee, G. Linares-Cruz, S. Fournier, and B. de Lingieres, "Influences of Percutaneous Administration of Estradiol and Progesterone on Human Breast Epithelial Cell Cycle in Vivo," *Fertility and Sterility 63 (1995) :785-791.*

11 T.S. Wiley, Julie Taguchi, M.D., Bent Formby, Ph.D., *Sex, Lies and Menopause,* 2003.

12 Becker, Jill B., et al. *Behavioral Endocrinology,* 1992, pgs. 58-59.

13 Collaborative Group on Hormonal Factors in Breast Cancer. Breast cancer and breastfeeding: collaborative reanalysis of individual data from 47 epidemiological studies in 30 countries, including 50,302 women with breast cancer and 96,973 women without the disease, *Lancet* 2002; 360:187-95.

14 Weiss, H, et al. *Epidemiology* 1997;8:181-7.

15 Formon, S., Infant feeding in the 20th century: formula and breast. *J Nutr* 2001 Feb;31(2): 409S-20S.

16 Mother's Survey, Ross Products Div. Abbott Labs, *Breastfeeding Trends 2002.*

17 *American Cancer Society.* Surveillance Research, 2001.

18 *FDA Consumer Magazine,* 1995.

19 Lemke, H, et al. Is there a maternally induced immunological imprinting phase? *Scand Immunol* 1999; 50:348-54.

20 *The John R. Lee Medical Letter,* July 1999, pg. 7.

21 Beral, V., Calle, E., *Cancer Research* UK, 2002.

22 *Harvard Medical Schools Consumer Health Information,* November, 2003.

23 Environmental Working Group, 2004.

24 http://www.lalecheleague.org/Release/contaminants.html - La Leche League International website, September 2003.

25 Williams, David G., *Alternatives for the Health-Conscious Individual,* Vol. 9, No. 22, April 2003.

26 Murray, Michael, N.D., Pizzorno, Joseph, N.D., *Encyclopedia of Natural Medicine,* 1998.

27 Lee, John R., M.D., *Optimal Health Guidelines* 1993.

28 Correa, P. 1981. Epidemiological correlations between diet and cancer frequency. *Cancer Res,* 41:3685-90.

29 National Dry Bean Council Undertakes Market Development Programs in Eastern Europe. *Northavest Bean Growers Association* May 2, 2003.

30 Choung, M. G., Choi, B. R., An, Y. N., Chu, Y. H., Cho, Y. S., Anthocyanin profile of Korean cultivated kidney bean. *J Agric Food Chem.* 2003, Nov 19;51(24):7040-3.

31 Rudin, D., MD and Felix, C., Omega-3 Oils 1996.

32 *American Journal of Clinical Nutrition*, 1999, 69:890-897.

33 *www.dukehealth.org Duke University Medical Center.*

34 Williams, David G., *Cures you can count on: New Breakthroughs Against Chronic Disease and Simple Steps to Great Daily Health*, 2000.

35 Lipski, E., M.S., C.C.N., *Digestive Wellness* 1996.

36 M. T. See and J. Odle, Effect of Dietary Fat Source, Level and Feeding Interval on Pork Fatty Acid Composition, 1998-2000 Departmental Report, *Department of Animal Science, ANS Report* No. 248 - North Carolina State University.

37 Lee, John R., M.D., *What Your Doctor May Not Tell You About Premenopause*, 1999.

38 Williams, David G., *Alternatives For The Health-Conscious Individual*, Vol. 8 February 2000.

39 Rackis, Joseph J. et al., "The USDA trypsin inhibitor study. I. Background, objectives and procedural details," *Qualification of Plant Foods in Human Nutrition*, Vol. 35, 1985.

40 www.drweil.com March 2004.

41 *Natural Medicine News* (L & H Vitamins, 32-33 47th Avenue, Long Island City, NY 11101), USA, January/February 2000, pg. 8.

42 Harras, Angela (ed.), *Cancer Rates and Risks*, National Institutes of Health, National Cancer Institute, 1996, 4th edition.

43 Ginsburg, Jean and Giordana M. Prelevic, "Is there a proven place for phytoestrogens in the menopause?" *Climacteric* (1999) 2:75-78.

44 FDA Reviews Health Claim Petition Regarding Reduction in Cancer Risk" *The Solae Company, Press Release, PR Newswire*, April 16, 2004.

45 Yamamoto, Y., Yamashita, S., Fujisawa, A., et al.: Oxidative stress in patients with hepatitis, cirrhosis, and hepatoma evaluated by plasma antioxidants. *Biochemical and Biophysical Research*

Communications 247(1): 166-170, 1998.

46 Yamamoto, Y., Yamashita, S.: Plasma ratio of ubiquinol and ubiquinone as a marker of oxidative stress. *Molecular Aspects of Medicine* 18 (suppl): S79-S84, 1997.

47 Lockwood, K., Moesgaard, S., Yamamoto, T., Folkers, K. Progress on therapy of breast cancer with vitamin Q10 and the regression of metastases. *Biochem Biophys Res Commun.* 1995 Jul 6;212(1):172-177.

48 Jolliet, P. et al, Plasma COQ10 concentrations in breast cancer: prognosis and therapeutic consequences. *Int J Clin Pharmacol Ther* 1998;36(9):506-509.

49 Chibo Hong, et. al. "Diindolylmethane (DIM), a dietary indole, has multiple cell suppressive effects on MCF-7, human breast cancer cells." *The American Society for Cell Biology,* Fortieth Annual Meeting, December 2000, San Francisco, California.

50 Wong, G. Y., et. al. "Dose-ranging study of indole-3-carbinol for breast cancer prevention." *J Cell Biochem Suppl* 1997; 28-29: 111-116.

51 "Safer Estrogen with Phytonutrition" *Townsend Letter for Doctors and Patients* (1999) April; 189:83-88.

52 Evans, Deborah, *Without Moral Limits,* 2000.

53 Fernandez, Jose, R., MD, The Pill vs. Natural Family Planning, www.onemoresoul.com 2004.

54 A. E. Washington, S. Gove, J. Schachter and R. L. Sweet, Oral contraceptives, Chlamydia trachomatis infection, and pelvic inflammatory disease. A word of caution about protection *JAMA,* Vol. 253 No. 15, April 19, 1985.

55 Null, Gary and Seaman, Barbara, *For Women Only! Your Guide to Health Empowerment,* Seven Stories Press, NY, 1999, p. 104.

56 Kemmeren, J., et al. Third generation oral contraceptives and risk of venous thrombo-disease: meta-analysis. *BJM* 2001;323: 1-9.

57 *The John R. Lee, M.D. Medical Letter,* October 2003 pg 3.

58 Gillum, L. A., Mamidipudi, S. K., and Johnston, S. C., Ischemic Stroke Risk With Oral Contraceptives. A Meta-Analysis, *JAMA* 2000; 284:72-78.

59 Oyelola, O., et al. Steroidal contraceptives and changes in individual plasma phospholipids: possible role in thrombosis. *Adv Contracept* 1990;6: 93-206.

60 Seaman, Barbara, et al. *Women and the Crisis in Sex Hormones.* Rawson Associates Publishers, Inc., New York, 1997. Page 83.

61 Kumle, M., et al. *JAMA,* October 11, 2002.

62 Newcomer, L. M., Newcomb, P. A., Trentham-Dietz, A., Longnecker, M. P., Greenberg, E. R., Oral contraceptive use and risk of breast cancer by histologic type *Int. J Cancer* 2003; 106:961-4.

63 *World Organization Ovulation Method Billings (WOOMB)* Proposed Statement to the 46TH Session Of The Commission On The Status Of Women - New York, March, 2002.

64 Hilgers, T. W. and Stanford, *J. Journal of Repro. Med.* 43: 495-502, June 1998.

65 Lawlor, D. A., Systematic Review of the Epidemiologic and Trial Evidence of an Association Between Antidepressant Medication and Breast Cancer. *Journal of Clinical Epidemiology.* 2003. Feb; 56(2): 155-163.

66 Moorman, P. G. et al. Antidepressant Medications and Their Association with Invasive Breast Cancer and Carcinoma in Situ of the Breast. *Epidemiology.* 2003. May; 14(3): 307-314.

67 Sharpe et al. The Effects of Tricyclic Antidepressants on Breast Cancer Risk. *British Journal of Cancer.* 2002 86(1): 92-97.

68 Cotterchio, M., et al. Antidepressant medication use and breast cancer risk. *Am J Epidemiol* 151(10):951-957.2000.

69 *Neuropsychopharmacology,* August 2001;25:277-289.

70 Lark, Susan., M.D., *The Lark Letter,* August 2003, pg. 8.

71 W.F. Byerley et al, "5-hydroxytryptophan: A Review of Its Antidepressant Efficacy and Adverse Effects," *J Clin Psychopharmacol* 7 (1987):127-37.

72 Peterson, C., Explanatory style as a risk factor for illness. *Cognitive Therapy and Research* 12 (1988):117-30.

73 Janet R. Daling et al.,"Risk of Breast Cancer Among Young Women: Relationship to Induced Abortion," 86 *Journal of the National Cancer Institute,* 1584, 1994.

74 Stewart et al. 1993 *J Clin Endocrinol Metab* 76:1470-6.

75 Witt et al. *Fertil Steril* 1990, 53:1029-36.

76 Kunz & Keller 1976 *Br J Ob Gyn* 83: 640-4.

77 Malec, Karen, president of the *Coalition on Abortion/Breast Cancer,* December 2004.

78 MacMahon et al. 1970 Bull Wld Health Org 43:209-21.

79 Brind et al. 1996 *J Epidemiol Community Health* 50: 481-96.

80 MacMahon et al. (1970) Bull Wld Health Org 43:209-21.

81 Beral V. Breast cancer and breastfeeding: collaborative re-analysis of individual data from 47 epidemiological studies in 30 countries, including 50,302 women with breast cancer and 96,973 women without the disease. *Lancet* 2002;360:187-195.

82 Graham Colditz, MD, "Relationship Between Estrogen Levels, Use of Hormone Replacement Therapy and Breast Cancer," *JNCI* (1998) 90:814-823.

83 Pike, M. C., Henderson BE, Casagrande JT, Rosario I, Gray GE. Oral contraceptive use and early abortion as risk factors for breast cancer in young women. *Br J Cancer*, 43:72-76.

84 *Journal of American Physicians and Surgeons* Vol. 8, Number 2, Summer 2003.

85 Foster, J., Abortion-cancer link goes to court, *World Net Daily*, August 26, 2000.

86 Byfield, J., Bearer of bad news: Alberta woman crashes a world conference with her message: abortion causes breast cancer. *Report News Magazine*, July 8, 2002.

87 Goodenough, P. First case linking abortion-breast cancer settled. *Cybercast News Service*, Jan 4, 2002.

88 Byrne, D., Why all the silence about abortion and breast cancer: *Chicago Tribune*, May 21, 2001, Sec. 1, pg. 17.

89 Byrne, D., Link between cancer, abortion: scientific evidence being ignored. *Chicago Tribune*, July 2, 2001, Sec. 1, pg. 13.

90 Pulliam, R., Politics and the neglected abortion-breast cancer link. *Indianapolis Star*, Sept.15, 2002, pg. D02.

91 Drake, T., Settlement on breast cancer may haunt abortion industry. *National Catholic Register*, Jan. 13-19, 2002, pg.1.

92 Mullan, F., Straight talk about US medicine. *Health Affairs* 2000; 19(1):117-123.

93 Dougherty, J., Can doctors be sued over abortion? Those who don't inform patients of breast-cancer link could be targets. *World Net Daily*, March 27, 2002.

94 *Agnes Bernardo, Pamela Colip, and Saundra Duffy-Hawkins v. Planned Parenthood Federation of American and Planned Parenthood of San Diego and Riverside Counties*, Superior Court of State of California, County of San Diego, Aug. 15, 2001.

95 Brind, J., Chinchilli, V. M., Severs, W. B., Summy-Long, J. Induced abortion as an independent risk factor for breast cancer: a comprehensive review and meta-analysis. *J Epidemiol Community Health* 1996;50:481-496.

96 Carroll, P., Trends and Risk Factors in English Breast Cancer. *British Journal of Cancer* 2004;91 (Suppl.1) S24(abstract).

CHAPTER 6: OSTEOPOROSIS . . . A PERSONAL STORY

1   The John R. Lee, M.D., *Medical Letter*, June 2002, pg. 5.

2   The Associated Press, Diagnoses Of Bone Thinning Proliferate, *Tampa Tribune*, July 2004.

3   *Nutrition Action Health Letter*, June 1993.

4   Murray, Michael, N.D. and Pizzorno, Joseph, N.D., *Encyclopedia of Natural Medicine*, Revised 2nd Edition, 1998.

5   Root, Leon., M.D., *Beautiful Bones Without Hormones*, 2004.

6   Veith, R., "Vitamin D supplementation, 25-hydroxyvitamin D concentrations, and safety." *Am J Clin Nutr* 1999;69:842-856.

7   *Pediatrics*, 2000, 106:40-44.

8   *Eur J Clin Nutr* 97;51(8):561-565.

9   *JAMA* 01;285(18):2323-2324.

10 Wiley, T. S., Taguchi, J., M.D., and Formby, B., Ph.D., *Sex, Lies, and Menopause*, 2003.

11 Lee, John R., M.D. and Hopkins, V., *What Your Doctor May Not Tell You About Menopause*, 1996.

12 Prior, J. C., Y. M. Vigna, and N. Alojado, Progesterone and the prevention of osteoporosis. *Canadian Journal of Obstetrics/Gynecology & Women's Health Care* 3:178-84.

13 Lee, John R., M.D., Hanley Jesse, M.D. and Hopkins, Virginia, *What Your Doctor May Not Tell You About Premenopause*, 1999.

14 Tom Lloyd, Vernon M. Chinchilli, Nan Johnson-Rollings, Kessey Kieselhorst, Douglas F. Eggli, and Robert Marcus., Adult Female Hip Bone Density Reflects Teenage Sports-Exercise Patterns But Not Teenage Calcium Intake, *PEDIATRICS* Vol. 106 No. 1 July 2000, pp. 40-44.

15 Surgeon General's Report on Bone Health, 2004.

16 Becker, Robert, O., M.D. *Body Electric: Electromagnetism and the Foundation of Life*, 1987.

17 Lark, Susan, M.D., *A Woman's Guide To Optimal Health &
    Balance*, May 2004.
18 J. Kanis. "Bone Density Measurements and Osteoporosis," *J Int
    Med* 241 (1997):173-75.
19 Chesnut, C. H., Hormone replacement therapy in post-
    menopausal women: urinary N-telopeptide of type I collagen
    monitors therapeutic effect and predicts response of bone mineral
    density. *Am J Med* 102(1): 29-37.

CHAPTER 7: THE HEART OF THE MATTER IS REVEALING

1 Statistics compiled from the National *Center on Health Statistics;
   National Heart, Lung and Blood Institute*; and *American Heart
   Association's 2005 Heart and Stroke Statistical Update.*
2 Hulley, S., Grady, D., Bush, T., et al. Randomized trial of
   estrogen plus progestin for secondary prevention of coronary
   heart disease in postmenopausal women. Heart and
   Estrogen/progestin Replacement Study (HERS) Research Group.
   Journal of the American Medical Association 1998;280(7):605-13.
3 Miyagawa, K., Rssch, J., Stanczyk, F., Hermsmeyer, K.,
   Medroxyprogesterone interferes with ovarian steroid protection
   against coronary vasospasm. *Nature Med.* 1997;3:324-327.
4 De Ziegler, D. Cardiovascular effects of the ovarian hormones.
   Arch Malad Coeur Vais 1996;89(suppl):9-16.
5 Jiang, C., Sarrel, P. M., Lindsay, D. C., Poole-Wilson, P. A.,
   Collins, P. Progesterone induces endothelium-independent relaxation of rabbit coronary artery in vitro. *Eur J Pharmacol.*
   1992;211:163-167.
6 Raloff J., Hormone Therapy: Issues of the Heart. *Science News.*
   1997;151;140. 3.
7 Williams, J. K., Adams, M. R., Estrogens, progestins and coronary
   artery reactivity. *Nature Med.* 1997;3:273-274.
8 Rosano, G., et al. Comparative cardiovascular effects of different
   progestins in menopause, *Int Fertil Womens Med* 2001; 46: 248-
   56.
9 Wiley, T. S., Taguchi, J. M.D., Formby, B. Ph.D., *Sex, Lies and
   Menopause*, 2003.
10 "Possible Peril Found in Menopause Cream," *New York Times*,

March 30, 2004.

11 Issue 4 *Hopkins Health Watch*, 2004.

12 Stephenson, Kenna, Price, Carol, Kurdowska, Anna et al., "Topical Progesterone Cream Does Not Increase Thrombotic and Inflammatory Factors in Postmenopausal Women," *Blood*, Volume 104, issue 11, November 16, 2004 .

13 Schwartz, D., Penckofer, S. Sex differences and the effects of sex hormones on homeostasis and vascular reactivity. *Heart Lung* 2001;30:401-26.

14 *Lancet.* 2001;357:1354-6.

15 Kawano, H., Motoyama, T., Ohgushi, M., Kugiyamam, K., Ogawa, H., Yasu, H., Menstrual cyclic variation of myocardial ischemia in premenopausal women with variant angina. *Ann Intern Med* 2001; 135:977-81.

16 Clin Sci (Lond) 1999;96:589-95.

17 Roysommuti, S., Khongnakha, T., Jirakulsomchok, D., Wyss, J. M., Excess dietary glucose alters renal function before increasing arterial pressure and inducing insulin resistance, *Am J Hypertens* 2002; 15:773-9.

18 Grant, W. B. Reassessing the role of sugar in the etiology of heart disease. *J Orthomolecular Med* 1998;13(2):95-104.

19 Wright, J.V., M.D., Preventing colds, flu and infection: Plan ahead to fight off germs for this fall's season of sickness. *Nutrition & Healing* 2001;8(4):1-3.

20 *Townsend Letter for Doctors and Patients*, January 2004, pgs. 102-103.

21 Hermsmeyer, K., Miyagawa, K., Kelley, S. T., Rosch, J., Hall, A.S., Axthelm, M. K., Greenberg, B. *J Am Coll Cardiol* 1997; 671-80.

22 Kloner, R. A., Jennings, R. B., Consequences of brief ischemia: stunning, preconditioning, and their clinical implications: part 2, *Circulation*, 2001 Dec 18;104(25):3158-67.

23 Richard D. Minshall, Frank Z. Stanczyk, Koichi, Miyagawa, Barry Uchida, Michael Axthelm, Miles Novy and Kent Hermsmeyer. Ovarian Steroid Protection Coronary Artery Hyperreactivity in Rhesus Monkeys, *J Clin Endocrinol Metab* 1998;83:649-659.

24 Ibid.

25 Ibid.

26 *The American Journal of the College of Nutrition*, 1997.

27 The *Lancet*, Volume 360, Issue 9346, 23 November 2002, Pages 1623-1630.

28 *The John R. Lee, M.D. Medical Letter*, June 2001, pg. 2.

29 The Dangers of Statin Drugs: What You Haven't Been Told About Cholesterol-Lowering Medication, Part I, www.mercola.com/2004/jul/21/statindrugs.htm

30 *The Low Carb Luxury Newsletter*, Vol. II, Issue, 15, August 2001.

31 Williams, D. G., Phillips Health, LLC, *Alternatives for the Health-Conscious Individual*, Special Report, 2001.

32 Lee, John R., M.D., *Commonsense Guide to a Healthy Heart* 1999.

33 University of Minnesota 1997.

34 Grimes, David A., Technology follies: the uncritical acceptance of medical innovations. *JAMA*. 1993;269:3030-3033.

35 Quick fixes for heart may not be best medicine, *St. Petersburg Times*, April 4, 2004.

36 Uffe, Ravnskov, MD, PhD. *The Cholesterol Myths*, New Trends Publishing, 2000.

37 Emery, Gene, *Reuters Health*, March 8, 2004,"More Potent Cholesterol Drugs Recommended".

38 Newman, T. B., Hulley, S. B., Carcinogenicity of lipid-lowering drugs, *JAMA* 1996;275:55-60.

39 Fassbender, K., Stroick, M., Bertsch, T., Ragoschke, A., Kuehl, S., Walter, S., Walter, J., Brechtel, K., Muehlhauser, F., Von Bergmann, K., Lutjohann, D., Effects of statins on human cerebral cholesterol metabolism and secretion of Alzheimer amyloid peptide. *Neurology* 2002;59(8): 1257-8.

40 "Bayer Voluntarily Withdraws Baycol," *U.S. Food and Drug Administration Talk*, August 8, 2001.

41 The Lipitor Dilemma, Smart Money: *The Wall Street Journal Magazine of Personal Business*, November 2003.

42 Jenkins, A. J., *BMJ* 2003 Oct 18;327(7420):933.

43 Krut, L. H., On the statins, correcting plasma lipid levels, and preventing the clinical sequelae of atherosclerotic coronary heart disease, *Am J Cardiol*,1998; April 15;81(8):1047-9.

44 *Circulation*, 2004 Feb 17;109(6):714-21.

45 *Tampa Tribune*, August 31, 2004.

46 Nissen, S. E., Not Just Lipid Levels, *JAMA*, August 2004.

47 Williams, D. G., Respectability for Sale, *Alternatives For The Health-Conscious Individual* Vol. 9, No.1, July 2001, pgs.1-3.

48 Williams, D. G., The Truth about cholesterol and the real cause of heart disease, *Alternatives For The Health-Conscious Individual Special Report*, Phillips Health, LLC, 2001.

49 Lee, John R., M.D.,*Optimal Health Guidelines*, 1993.

50 Udo, Erasmus, *Fats That Kill and Fats that Heal*, 1994, pg. 253.

51 M. Trevisan, V. Krogh, J. Freudenheim, A. Blake, P. Muti, S. Panico, E. Farinaro, M. Mancini, A. Menotti and G. Ricci, Consumption of olive oil, butter, and vegetable oils and coronary heart disease risk factors. *JAMA*, 263:5, February 2, 1990: 688-691.

52 D. T. Nash; S. D. Nash, State University of New York Health Science Center, Syracuse, NY, *Journal of the American College of Cardiology*, 925-116, 1993.

53 D. T. Nash, State University of New York Health Science Center, Syracuse, NY: *Arteriosclerosis*, an Official Journal of the American Heart Association, Vol. 10, No. 6, Nov-Dec. 1990.

54 Peat, R., Ph.D., *From PMS to Menopause: Female Hormones in Context*, 1997.

55 I. A. Prior, F. Davidson, C. E. Salmond, Z. Czochanska. "Cholesterol, coconuts, and diet on Polynesian atolls: a natural experiment: the Pukapuka and Tokelau island studies." *Am J Clin Nutr.* 1981 Aug; 34(8):1552-61.

56 Kang, J. X, Leaf, A. Anti-arrhythmic effects of polyunsaturated fatty acids. *Circulation* 1996;94:1774–80.

57 Bang, H. O., Dyerberg, J., The composition of food consumed by Greenlandic Eskimos. *Acta Med Scand* 1973;200:69–73.

58 Dyerberg, J., Bang, H. O. Haemostatic function and platelet polyunsaturated fatty acids in Eskimos. *Lancet* 1979;2:433–5.

59 Lark, Susan M., M.D., *Nutritional Supplementation*, 2002.

60 Sakai, M., et al. "Experimental studies on the role of fructose in the development of diabetic complications." *Kobe J Med Sci.* 2002 Dec; 48(5-6): 125-136.

61 Beatrice Trum Hunter, "Confusing Consumers About Sugar Intake," *Consumers Research*, 78, No. 1 (January 1995): 14-17.

62 *The John R. Lee, M.D. Medical Letter*, pgs.1-2, May 2002.

63 Isokangas, P., Alanen, P., Tiekso, J., et al. Xylitol chewing gum in caries prevention: a field study in children. *J Am Dent Assoc.* 1988;117:315-320.

64 Uhari, M., Kontiokari, T., Koskela, M., Niemela, M. Xylitol chewing gum in prevention of acute otitis media: double blind randomized trial. *Br Med J* (1996) 313:1180-1184.

65 *Anon.* "Stevia components as sweetening agents and antibiotics." Japanese Patent #8092,323. 1980.

66 Blumenthal, Mark. "Perspectives on FDA's new stevia policy, after four years, the agency lifts its ban—but only partially." *Whole Foods Magazine*, February 1996.

67 Hunter, B. T. Sucralose. *Consumers' Research Magazine*, Oct. 1990, Vol. 73 Issue 10, p8, 2p.

68 *Townsend Letter for Doctors and Patients*- August/September 2004, pgs. 119-121.

69 Roger J. Williams, Ph.D., A World-Renowned Biochemist Specializing in Nutrition, Biochemical Individuality, and Public Education.

70 Stavroula, Osganian, M.D., Balz Frei, M.D., Vitamin C Cuts Heart Disease Risk in Women, *Journal of the American College of Cardiology*, July 16, 2003.

71 *National Research Council: Recommended Dietary Allowances*, 10th edition. National Academy Press, Washington, D.C., 1989.

72 Sesso, H. D., Buring, J. E., Norkus, E. P., Gaziano, J. M. "Plasma lycopene, other carotenoids, and retinol and the risk of cardiovascular disease in women." *Am J Clin Nutr* 2004 ;79 (1): 47-53.

73 Sesso, H. D., Liu, S., Gaziano, J. M., Buring, J. E. "Dietary lycopene, tomato-based food products and cardiovascular disease in women." *J Nutr* 2003; 133(7): 2336-2341.

74 Weber, C., Bysted, A., and Holmer, G.: The coenzyme Q10 content of the average Danish diet. *Int J Vit Nutr Res* 1997;67:123-9.

75 Weber, C., et al.: Effect of dietary coenzyme Q10 as an antioxidant in human plasma. *Mol Aspects Med* 1994;15 (Suppl.):s 97-102.

76 Folkers, K., Vadhanavikit, S. and Mortensen, S. A.: Biochemical rationale and myocardial tissue data on the effective therapy of cardiomyopathy with coenzyme Q10. *Proc Natl Acad Sci* 1985;82:901.

77 Ibid.

78 Langsjoen, H., et al.: Usefulness of coenzyme Q10 in clinical cardiology: a long-term study. *Mol Aspects Med* 1994;15(Suppl.):s165-75.

79 Sinatra, Stephen T., M.D., *Heart Sense for Women*, 2000.

CHAPTER 8: THE FINAL ANALYSIS . . .
PUTTING IT ALL INTO PERSPECTIVE

1   Grange, John, M., *The Owl and the Pussy Cat put to Sea: Science and Holism in the New Millennium*. Address to the London Medical Society, May 1999.

2   Stephenson, Joan, Ph.D., Exposure to Home Pesticides Linked to Parkinson Disease *JAMA*. 2000; 283:3055-3056.

3   *Curr Opin Neurol* 00;13(6):687-90).

4   Ritz, B., Yu, F., Parkinson's disease mortality and pesticide exposure in California 1984-1994. *Int J Epidemiol* 2000;29:323-9.

5   *Tampa Tribune*, Associated Press, July 14, 2002.

6   Winter, Ruth, M.S., *A Consumer's Dictionary of Cosmetic Ingredients*, 1991.

7   Hampton, Aubrey, *Natural Ingredients Dictionary*.

8   *Prevention is the Cure, Cancer Risk Reduction, Breast Cancer options, Inc.*, www.breastcanceroptions.org

9   Lark, Susan, M.D., *The Lark Letter*, June 2004, pgs. 2-5.

10 *The John R. Lee, M.D. Medical Letter*, October 2003, pgs. 5-6.

11 Lee, John R., M.D., Zava, D., PhD., Hopkins, V, *What Your Doctor May Not Tell You About Breast Cancer*, 2002.

12 Amid Health Concern, Nail-Polish Makers Switch Formulas, *Wall Street Journal*, April 2004.

13 Dispenza, Joseph, *Live Better Longer: The Parcells Center 7-Step Plan for Health and* Longevity, 2000.

14 *American Journal of Industrial Medicine* Vol. 39, Issue 2, 2001.

SUGGESTED READINGS

BOOKS

What Your Doctor May Not Tell You About Breast Cancer
> John R. Lee, M.D., David Zava, PhD. and Virginia Hopkins

What Your Doctor May Not Tell You About Menopause
> John R. Lee, M.D.

What Your Doctor May Not Tell You About Premenopause
> John R. Lee, M.D., Jesse Hanley, M.D. and Virginia Hopkins

Hormone Balance For Men
> John R. Lee, M.D.

Optimal Health Guidelines
> John R. Lee, M.D.

Manifesto For A New Medicine
> James S. Gordon, M.D.

Stress Management (21st Century Health and Wellness)
> James S. Gordon, M.D. and C. Everett Koop, M.D.

Health for the 21st Century...cellular health series
> Matthias Rath, M.D.

Hormone Replacement Therapy -YES or NO?
> Betty Kamen, PhD.

A Woman's Guide to a Healthy Heart
> Carol Simontacchi, CCN, MS

Preventing and Reversing Osteoporosis
> Alan, Gaby, M.D.

Heart Sense for Women
> Stephen T. Sinatra, M.D.

The Breast Cancer Prevention Program
> Samuel S. Epstein, M.D. and David Steinman

The Politics of Cancer Revisited
> Samuel S. Epstein, M.D.

Cancer-Gate
> Samuel S. Epstein, M.D.

Breast Cancer Prevention Diet
    Bob Arnot, M.D.
Encyclopedia of Natural Medicine
    Michael, Murray, N.D. and Joseph Pizzorno, N.D.
The Complete System of Self-Healing Internal Exercises
    Stephen T. Chang, M.D.
Nutrition for Women
    Raymond Peat, Ph.D.
Toxic Relief
    Don Colbert, M.D.
Adrenal Fatigue: The 21st Century Stress Syndrome
    James L. Wilson, N.D., D.C., Ph.D.
The Real Vitamin and Mineral Book
    Shari Lieberman, Ph.D.
What The Bible Says About Healthy Living
    Rex Russell, M.D.
Smart Medicine for a Healthier Child
    Janet Zand, LAc OMD, Rachel Walton R.N,
    and Robert Rountree, M.D.
The Hysterectomy Hoax
    Stanley West, MD
Live Better Longer
    Joseph Dispenza
Sex, Lies, and MENOPAUSE
    T. S. Wiley, Julie Taguchi, M.D. and Bent Formby, Ph.D.
Seven Keys to Vibrant Health
    Terry Lemerond, 3rd Edition
The Billings Method - Using the body's natural signal of fertility to
    achieve or avoid pregnancy, New Edition 2003
    Dr. Evelyn Billings & Dr. Ann Westmore
Trust Us, We're Experts: How Industry Manipulates Science and
    Gambles With Your Future
    Sheldon Rampton and John Stauber
Apple Cider Vinegar-Miracle Health System
    Paul C. Bragg, N.D., Ph.D, and Patricia Bragg, N.D., Ph.D.
Menstrual Cramps: A Self Help Program
    Susan M. Lark, M.D.

Home Safe Home
Debra Lynn Dadd

NEWSLETTERS

Nutrition & Healing
Jonathan V. Wright, M.D. 203.699.3683
Alternatives For The Health Conscious Individual
David G. Williams, DC 800.527.3044
The HERS (Hysterectomy Educational Resources and Services)
Nora Coffey, President Foundation 610.667.7757
Health & Healing
Dr. Julian Whitaker 800.539.8219
The Lark Letter – A Women's Guide To Optimal Health & Balance
Susan Lark, M.D. 877.437.5275
HOW-Health Opportunities for Women
877.547.5499

JOURNALS/MAGAZINES

Townsend Letter for Doctors & Patients
360.385.6021
Alternative Medicine
800.333.HEAL
Alternative Therapies in Health and Medicine
800.345.8112

OTHER INFORMATIVE RESOURCES

People Against Cancer, provides a comprehensive counseling service
called the Alternative Therapy Program. It includes a review of your
medical records by a network of doctors using alternative therapies. It
costs $250. People Against Cancer can be reached at 515.972.4444.
http://www.peopleagainstcancer.net

The Ralph Moss Reports contain a critical overview of the latest
conventional therapies for all types of cancers as well as a focus on
what they believe to be the most worthwhile complementary and
alternative (CAM) treatments. The conventional sections of many of

the reports on the most common cancers have now been revised. They contain discussions of the latest research on the various diseases, culled from the world's scientific databases as well as their own sources. To schedule a phone consult or request a report from the U.S. call 800.980.1234 or from abroad call 814.238.3367. www.cancerdecisions.com

Vitamin Companies and Products

BioActive Nutrients
1300 Roundhouse Rd.
Spooner, WI 54801
800.879.6504
www.bioactivenutrients.com

VAXA, International
4010 State Street
Tampa, FL 33609
888.278.3771

Metagenics
100 Ave. La Pata
San Clemente, CA 92673
800.692.9400

Enzymatic Therapies
Green Bay, WI 54311
800.783.2286

Dr. David Williams
Mountain Home Nutritionals
800.888.1415

Susan Lark, M.D.
Daily Balance, Inc.
P.O. Box 3100
Forrester Center, WV 25438-9948
888.314.5275

Mathias Rath, M.D., Inc.
2901 Bayview Drive
Fremont, CA 94538
888.827.8700

North Star Nutritionals
Allan Spreen, M.D., Hyla Cass, M.D., Arnold J. Susser, R.P., Ph.D.
P.O. Box 925
Frederick, MD 21705
800.311.1950

Standard Process
1200 West Royal Lee Drive
Palmyra, WI 53156
262.495.6451

Some Favorite Websites

Preservion, Inc. – www.preservion.com

John R. Lee – www.johnleemd.com

Power Surge - www.power-surge.com

Progesterone Benefits by Dr. R.H. Logan,
        Instructor of Chemistry, North Lake College, Irving, TX
        www.members.aol.com/profchm/rahman.html

Citizens for Health: Defending Your Right to Choose
        www.citizens.org

ConsumerLab.com - Best quality health and nutrition products
        are identified through independent testing.
        http://www.consumerlab.com - 914.722.9149

American Holistic Health Association (AHHA)
        www.ahha.org - 714.779.6152

American College for Advancement in Medicine (ACAM)
        www.acam.org 800.532.3688 or 949.583.7666

Health Sciences Institute – www.HSIBaltimore.com

Healing Edge Sciences - www.healingedge.net

All Organic Links -The Global Resource for Organic Information
http://www.allorganiclinks.com/

American Academy of Environmental Medicine (AAEM)
www.aaem.com - 316.684.5500

American Holistic Medical Association
www.holisticmedicine.org - 703.556.9245

American Association of Naturopathic Physicians
www.naturopathic.org - 866.538.2267

American Osteopathic Association - www.aoa-net.org - 800.621.1773

Breast Cancer Prevention - http://www.bcpinstitute.org/home.htm

Coalition on Abortion/Breast Cancer
http://www.abortionbreastcancer.com

The Leading Cancer Treatment Information Resource
http://www.cancerdecisions.com/index.html

Lorraine Day, M.D. - Natural, Alternative Therapies for all Diseases,
including Cancer and AIDS,
http://www.drday.com/index2.htm

Dr. Matthias Rath's Health Alliance – A grassroots movement
designed to educate and encourage consumers to take
control of their health. – www.drrathresearch.org

Jonathan V. Wright, M.D. medical clinic
http://www.tahoma-clinic.com/index.shtml

Natural approaches to fertility - http://www.naprotechnology.com

Shari Lieberman, Ph.D., research scientist and clinician
http://www.drshari.net

Susan M. Lark, M.D., the foremost authority in the field of clinical
nutrition and preventive medicine-www.drlark.com

Vital Health Publishing - Experts answer questions related to food
and environmental issues that affect your health.
http://www.foodintegrity.com

WholeHealth M.D. – Empowers consumers to take a proactive
approach to wellness and is dedicated to providing the
best of integrative and wellness solutions.
www.wholehealthmd.com

PROGESTERONE CREMES

FemCreme
Pure Essence Laboratories, Inc.
P.O. Box 95397
LasVegas, NV 89193
888.254.8000

Fem-Gest
Bio-Nutritional Formulas
106 East Jericho Turnpike
Mineola, NY 11501
800.950.8484

Preserve For Women
VAXA, International
4010 State Street
Tampa, FL   33609
888.278.3771

Progestacare Cream
Life-flo Health Care Products
8146 North 23 Avenue, Suite E
Phoenix, AZ 85021
888.999.7440

The Natural Hormone Institute of America
Dr. Randolph's Natural Progesterone Cream
1891 Beach Boulevard, Suite 100
Jacksonville, FL 32250
904.694.0037

Vitamin Research Products, Inc.
HerBalance Cream
3579 Highway 50 East
Carson City, NV 89701
775.884.1300 or 800.877.2447

Saliva Hormone Testing

ZRT Laboratory
1815 NW 168th Place, Suite 5050
Beaverton, OR 97006
503.466.2445
www.salivatest.com

Hormone Hotline: 503.466.9166
24-hour taped audio-library with a growing list of topics on every
aspect of hormone balance and testing.
View the available auditory list.

Mead Labs, LLC
Saliva Testing and Consultations
Jay H. Mead MD, pathologist, FASCP, ACAM and Medical Director
4444 SW Corbett Ave.
Portland, OR 97239
Order hotline: 503.546.0800
Questions: info@meadlabs.com

Other Great Natural Products and Resources

Honey Bee Skin Healing Cream
The Link Group, Inc.
P.O. Box 22386
Orlando, FL 32830
407.238.1375
www.honeybeez.com

Natural Beauty Products
Cosmetics Without Synthetics (CWS), Inc.
P.O. Box 701
Dewey, AZ 86327
888.586.9719
www.allnaturalcosmetics.com

Aubrey Organics
4419 N. Manhattan Ave.
Tampa, FL 33614
800.282.7394
www.aubrey-organics.com

Jason Natural Cosmetics
5500 W. 83rd St.
Los Angeles, CA 90045
Toll Free: 877.JASON-01 ext. 102

Avalon Natural Products
1105 Industrial Ave., Suite 2
Petaluma, CA 94952
800.742.5841

Environmental Media Services- Environmentally friendly products and
alternatives to commercial cleaners and other household products
1320 18th Street NW 5th Floor
Washington, DC 20036
202.463.6670

Natural Alternatives to Pesticides
Gardens Alive – www.gardens-alive.com
Andy Lopez – www.invisiblegardener.com
EcoPCO – www.ecosmart.com

For Wet Cleaning Clothes
    www.Checnet.org

La Leche League International - breast-feeding information
    800.LA-LECHE or 847.519.7730.

For more information on Natural Family Planning:
Billings Ovulation Method Assn-USA
    651.699.8139 www.Boma-usa.org
The Couple To Couple League (STM)

513.471-2000 www.ccli.org
Family of the Americas Foundation
301.627.3346 www.familyplanning.net
Northwest Family Services (STM)
503.215.6377 www.nwfs.org
Pope Paul VI Institute
402.390.6600 www.popepaulvi.com
One More Soul
800.307.7685 www.OMSoul.com
FertilityCare™ Services of Tampa Bay
813.839.6803

PRACTITIONER RESOURCES

American College for Advancement in Medicine
(ACAM) – 800.532.3688, 949.583.7666, www.acam.org - can
provide a list of doctors near you who are skilled in natural medicine.
ACAM is a not-for-profit association of physicians in various fields
who believe in using natural alternatives in their practice. Their
website listing will also indicate if the doctor has a specialty - some
specialize in bio-identical hormone replacement.

American Association of Naturopathic Physicians (AANP).
www.naturopathic.org - listing of qualified naturopathic doctors
(N.D.s) in your area. N.D.s take a wholistic approach to health,
looking at the entire person, not just a subset of symptoms.

Holistic Healthcare Website: www.healers.com

Tahoma Clinic
Jonathan V. Wright, M.D.
801 SW 16th
Renton, WA 98055
425.264.0059
Dedicated to promoting the enormous potential of nutritional therapy
and natural medicine. **The 2/16 ratio test is available through the
Tahoma Clinic and Meridian Valley Laboratory (425.271.8689).

Joseph M. Mercola, D.O.
1443 W. Schaumburg Road, Suite 250
Schaumburg, IL 60194
847.985.1777

Nutrition for Optimal Health Association
P.O. Box 380
Winnetka, IL 60093
www.nutrition4health.org
847.60HEALTH (847.604.3258)
NOHAinfo@aol.com

FLORIDA PHYSICIAN RESOURCES

Ignacio Armas, M.D.
OB/GYN
425 S. Parsons, Suite 101,
Brandon, FL 33511
813.681.6625

Ron Schemesh, M.D.
Natural Health Center
OB/GYN
14372 N. Dale Mabry Hwy.
Tampa, FL 33618
813.935.2273
Energy Work and more.

Gael Wheeler, D.O. and Douglas Nelson, D.O.
Carrollwood Integrative Medicine
16622 N. Dale Mabry Hwy.
Tampa, FL 33618
813.265.8885

Carol Roberts, M.D.
Wellness Works
1209 Lakeside Drive
Brandon, FL 33510
813.661.3662
www.wellnessworks.us

Karen L. Mutter, D.O., P.A.
Board Certified/Internal Medicine
Integrative Medicine Healing Center
5770 Roosevelt Blvd., Suite 300
Clearwater, FL 33760
727.524.0900

C. W. Randolph, Jr., M.D.
The Natural Hormone Institute of America
1891 Beach Boulevard, Suite 100
Jacksonville, FL 32250
904.694.0037

Don Colbert, M.D.
Divine Health Wellness Center
Cambridge Square Office Park
1908 Boothe Circle
Longwood, FL 32750
407.331.7007

INDEX

PRESERVION, INC.

Preservion, Inc. is your comprehensive and well researched guide to the best healthcare information, resources and alternatives.

Cindy A. Krueger, M.P.H., President and Founder of Preservion, Inc. provides research, consultation and education services that are intended to provide clients with timely and well researched information from researchers, health practitioners and scientists who support the efforts of integrative and natural approaches to health and healing.

When it comes to the health and safety of consumers, there is no such thing as a calculated risk. Consumers need to make good informed healthcare decisions.

Count on Preservion, Inc. to:

- personalize healthcare strategies that focus on prevention and healing and move away from solely curative treatment that directly affects productivity and quality of life issues,
- assist clients with a working knowledge of where to find and how to use good healthcare information,
- customize healthcare strategies and assist clients in learning how to use their healthcare dollars most effectively and efficiently, and
- conduct engaging presentations that challenge the audience to think critically about the risk/benefit ratio of healthcare interventions.

Contact Preservion, Inc. for more information at consulting@preservion.com or call 813.289.9282.